AN UNTOLD MEDICAL STORY

CORONARY BLOOD FLOW, HEART ATTACK PREDICTION, PREVENTION AND TREATMENT

By

Gunnar Sevelius, MD

AuthorHouse™
1663 Liberty Drive
Bloomington, IN 47403
www.authorhouse.com
Phone: 1-800-839-8640

First published by AuthorHouse 4/8/2011

ISBN: 978-1-4567-4890-6 (e)
ISBN: 978-1-4567-4891-3 (dj)
ISBN: 978-1-4567-4892-0 (sc)

Library of Congress Control Number: 2011904361

Printed in the United States of America

Any people depicted in stock imagery provided by Thinkstock are models, and such images are being used for illustrative purposes only. Certain stock imagery © Thinkstock.

This book is printed on acid-free paper.

OTHER BOOKS BY THE AUTHOR

In English:
Add Years to Your Life and Life to Your Years
Part I. Heart Attack Prevention

Add Years to Your Life and Life to Your Years
Part II. Family and Work Enhancement

You Are It: First Aid

Radioisotopes and Circulation, Editor

The Nine Pillars of History
Also a Guide for Peace

The Nine Pillars of History
An Anthropological Review of History, Five Religions, Sexuality and
Modern Economics, All as a Guide for Peace

In Swedish:
Historiens Nio Grundstenar
Även en Guide för Fred

DEDICATION

This report is published in memory of Professor Stewart Wolf, Chief of Medicine at the University of Oklahoma.

Professor Wolf was my professor in Medicine. He relentlessly supported me and made the following work possible.

INTRODUCTION

Medical research is the weaving of a tapestry; different information needs to be woven together to create a complete picture. The work of predicting heart attacks with help of the radiocardiogram in the 1950s and 1960s was halted by life's circumstances and left a hole in the tapestry.

This publication is written from old notes and memory. The purpose of this publication is to collect the different published and non-published reports of my work with the radiocardiogram and to explain the purpose of the different steps. I hope some young scientist will be inspired to pick up the work with the radiocardiogram because I still believe it has a lot to offer medicine in general.

The first step would be to establish blood flow in a depressed patient with resistant heart failure. What needs to be done is to establish his or her optimal cardiac output and blood volume from the standpoint of circulatory efficiency, that is, from the strength of the heart muscle vs. the size of the blood volume instead of vs. the body size. From then on lies a new open field of blood rheology for numerous physical and mental circulatory conditions as well as the evaluation of the efficacy of drugs in these conditions.

My unique experiences with health education, its efficacy in a large working population, may also be useful information.

ACKNOWLEDGEMENTS

My thanks to Roger Potash, engineer expert in fluid dynamics and retired colleague and friend from Lockheed years, for reviewing my comments about Poiseuilles' Law.

As always, I am thankful to the dedicated mother and daughter team, Cheryl Cooper and Wendi Freeman, for formatting and editing the manuscript into digital form.

TABLE OF CONTENTS

PART I
Can Blood Flow be Measured
Through the Skin?

Stockholm, 1955
A Medical Idea

A common medical complication during pregnancy is so called "toxemia of pregnancy." It is characterized by high blood pressure, gain of weight, and protein in the urine. It is most common in obese women.

The idea was that the growing fetus within the uterus was dominating in its demand for blood, causing the kidneys to be hungry for oxygen. A blood-hungry kidney cannot do its work normally. The kidney will let protein from the blood through to the urine and may raise blood pressure to relieve its oxygen hunger. In obese women, not only the uterus but also the extra fat would lower the margin for blood available to the kidney.

I had to work within the field of obstetrics in order to pursue the idea. There was a job opening at a large women's clinic in Stockholm. I was 27 years old and worked as a licensed physician for the first time.

At the time, I was reading about measuring blood flow by marking the bloodstream with a bolus of isotope and recording its flow with a detector placed over the skin. It might be informative to record a change in blood flow to the kidney versus to the uterus in toxemia of pregnancy.

In 1948, Dr. M. Prinzmetal, the inventor of surface scanning, named a recording from the heart area a "radiocardiogram." The marker of the blood was an isotope Iodine-131 bound to a simple blood albumin. Circumstances would have me work with the radiocardiogram for the next 13 years.

For different reasons my publications on the subject are spread to sites not easily accessible. The purpose of this publication is to collect all the publications of this work into one place. The scientific reports constitute the appendix to this publication and act as the background to my personal story. The overall purpose is to promote the radiocardiogram as a simple technique to evaluate the efficiency of the heart, the basic energy source for the total body all through life.

The Chief of Medicine, Dr. Lars Werko, came for weekly medical consultations to the Department of Obstetrics. He listened to my idea about toxemia of pregnancy. He arranged for me to go to the United States for a year as a first-year resident in Internal Medicine. This was a deviation from my interest in OB/GYN and surgery. My classmate/colleague, Hilli, who was now also my wife, and I figured we would make the best of it just for the fun of visiting the USA.

Oklahoma City, 1956
From Kidney Flow to Coronary Flow

At the end of September, I reported in to Professor Stewart Wolf, Chief of Medicine at the University of Oklahoma Medical School. I told Professor Wolf about my wife graduating three months after me. He answered, "Ask Hilli to come over when she has graduated." Hilli arrived at Christmas. Both of us enrolled in a First Year Residency in Internal Medicine.

My wife was three months behind me in her residency year and I was free for three months. Dr. Phillip C. Johnson, a very dynamic and open personality, was Chief of the Radioisotope Laboratory at the Veterans Hospital in Oklahoma City. He listened to my ideas about scanning the bloodstream.

In 1955 Dr. Huff et al. had reported that he had a formula to calculate the cardio output (CO), the total amount of blood the heart pumps per minute, using the Prinzmetal radiocardiogram.

The CO was simply blood volume (BV) times the ratio between the equilibrium recording (E) (the follow-up steady state recording when the total blood volume was homogenously mixed with the isotope) and the area (A) under the flow curve.

$$CO = E/A \times BV \times 3$$

where 3 stood for a correction for the different units involved in the calculation.

Dr. Huff et al. had never explained why his formula worked and neither had anybody else. BV was not a part of the regular dye formula for the calculation of cardiac output. The dye formula was a pure time/concentration curve calibrated directly in the sensors for the recording and with no factor dependent on BV.

Dr. Johnson picked out what I needed from his large isotope laboratory. His laboratory occupied almost a full story of the Veterans Hospital. We would start with placing two detectors, one over each kidney. The radiation exposure was minimal (that is, 20% of a chest x-ray's 30 mrad or about a total of 6 mrad). A veteran volunteered.

Soon, I sat at a desk looking at a long wiggly curve. Which of the wiggles represented the bolus passing through the kidneys and were not simply scintillations from the isotope? I had to know when the blood reached the kidney in order to at least know when the kidney blood flow started.

I got an idea. I would mix the isotope solution with a mixture that tasted bad. When the patient felt a bad taste in the mouth the isotope had also reached the kidney. Blood moves very quickly in the bloodstream; the time from the arm to the tongue is usually around 16 seconds. The difference between the arrival times to the kidney and the tongue would be minimal or fractions of seconds. When the patient felt a bad taste, the recording indeed started a larger peak.

This was the time in medicine when kidney transplants were sensational. A veteran with a non-working left kidney was admitted to the hospital. I was asked to do a flow curve over each kidney. I showed the recordings to Professor Wolf on a Saturday morning. There was no doubt that one could see the difference in the curves from each kidney area. While looking at the recordings Professor Wolf said, "Gunnar, you stay here and do this."

Monday morning I had a lab to work in and the head technician, Dan Patrick, to help me.

Organ flow can change in two ways, either by increased flow from the heart or by opening the arteries locally to an organ. Things started to become complicated. I had to know what happened in the heart at the same time as I recorded what was happening in the kidneys. I had to have three channels and also to know the relative sensitivity between the different channels.

Luckily, the lab was full of isotope machines. I went down to the lumberyard, bought some 4x4 posts, and built stands for all the scanners.

We changed the time delay in the recorders so the curves smoothed out the isotope scintillations. A 0.3 second time delay smoothed out scintillation wiggles and gave a representative picture of the blood flowing by.

The heart curve had two peaks, one for the isotope going through the right heart and one when it came back from the lungs and went through the left heart. Dr. Huff et al. had worked with a one-peak curve, supposedly sampling the isotope marker from a singular artery, similarly to those who used to measure cardiac output with a dye.

A dye curve required an arterial sampling. Huff's improvement would be that his technique would save the patient from an arterial puncture, a painful procedure and sometimes with complications.

We now recorded flow curves from the heart, each kidney, and marked when the patient felt a bitter taste in the mouth. A flow curve rises very quickly as the "head" of bolus comes in under the detector and has always an exponentially falling tail as the tail of the bolus passes by.

We sometimes noticed a break in the otherwise smooth exponentially fall of the tail from the left heart curve when the patient would scream out "#*&!" Could this be the third chamber in the heart, the one from the coronary circulation? Coronary flow is only 5% of the heart flow but isotopes cannot hide from this kind of very sensitive detectors.

I showed the curves to Professor Wolf. His answer was, "Gunnar, this would be more important than kidney flow. Change your goal and explore coronary flow instead."

This was Dr. Wolf's way of making decisions. He did not care much about formalities. This would catch up with both Hilli and I. Neither of us had a medical license to work independently in the State of Oklahoma.

Our employment during residency was allowed for training purposes under licensed supervision. A doctor could work in a laboratory without direct responsibility for the care of a patient. These rules were the same throughout the United States.

Hilli finished her residency in Internal Medicine and was offered a fellowship in gastroenterology and later in drug efficacy. I received a First Prize from the staff for my research in 1958. This was repeated in 1959 and 1960.

Professor Wolf thought we should report the findings to the National Conference of Medicine in Atlantic City. Medical research is always first reported locally, and then to one of four regional meetings—the west, north, south and east United States. The most interesting works are selected for a national meeting in the spring in Atlantic City and the most significant are selected for its general first day morning session. Our report was selected for the Atlantic City general morning session. Thousands of the world's most experienced medical scientists were present.

This was my first medical presentation. I practiced in front of several department heads in our medical center and presented my curves in Atlantic City.

A doctor from Seattle, where Dr. Huff worked, said he had never seen a double-hump radiocardiogram, and certainly not a three-peaked one. I doubted he had scanned the heart because the bolus had to pass under the counter three times. This was an anatomical fact.

Never did I imagine that I would spend the next 12 years working on how to split up the heart curve into its three parts.

A German, Dr. Adolph Fick, had invented the first method to measure cardiac output in 1870. He worked on horses using a gas. The gas would clear from the body through the lungs depending on how fast the heart pumped the blood. This is called a clearance technique. Fifty years later, in 1921, an American, G.N. Stewart, invented a dye formula for the measuring of blood flow. The dye technique is based on marking the venous blood with a bolus of dye as it flows towards the right heart and sampling an artery after the bolus has left the left side of the heart. A recorder records the concentration of the dye for each unit of time as it passes through the artery. The sensitivity of the recorder has to be calibrated but otherwise the area under the concentration/time curve is inversely proportional to the flow rate or the Cardiac Output (CO).

Different dyes or markers have been used and Iodine-131 isotope would be just one other dye. The surface recording would save the patient from the arterial puncture.

Both the Fick and the Stewart techniques have been used in medical research but have had relatively little breakthrough in clinical medicine. Results were normalized for the size of the person. The size of the person came from a normogram based on the person's height, weight and a "factor" yielding an estimate of the surface area of the body. The determined CO was divided or normalized with the person's body surface area to yield what is called Cardiac Index (CI). The CI was used for the clinical assessment of the CO.

The CI hardly gave any better assessment of the patient's heart condition than a clinical exam by an experienced cardiologist. I did not know this at the time but in laboratory terms this means that the standard deviations of the results were too wide to be clinically effective. CI had just too many false positive and false negative results.

Physical Evidence of Coronary Blood Flow

A new technique requires a confirmation. The Chief of the Surgical Department at our Veterans Administration (V.A.) Hospital assigned a surgical resident, Dr. David Snider, to work with me. David was going to either temporarily occlude the two coronary arteries with two snares or have the coronaries have a separate perfusion from the femoral arteries, while I recorded a radiocardiogram. I designed a special collimator, a cone-shaped piece of lead with a one-inch front opening, to monitor the heart through the chest of a dog. The heart kept on beating, undisturbed, for the less than seven seconds the bolus was passing through the coronaries.

Two curves were recorded, one with the coronaries open and one with the coronaries closed, or separately perfused from the femoral arteries. The coronary part of the radiocardiogram was very large when coronaries were open and disappeared when they were closed. Not only did the coronary peaks disappear but the washout from the left curve went down almost to the baseline. (See Figure 1.)

This indicated that the coronary flow was by far the fastest in the body. The coronary blood is squeezed through the heart muscle each time the heart contracts. The washout curve from the left heart alone was pure logarithmic. This would speak for the fact that we had isolated the coronary circulation and that radiation from the chest wall and other close-by organs were very small. David reported the results in the *Journal of Surg., Gynec. & Obst.* in 1960. This was qualitative proof that the coronary flow was part of the radiocardiogram.

I needed a quantitative amount of blood flow through the coronaries for a clinical measurement to be useful.

My first inclination was simply to try to separate the third peak using a French curve. I soon realized this would get me nowhere. (Dr. Johnson eventually left Oklahoma City to lead an isotope laboratory at Baylor Medical Center in Houston. From here he reported that he also had no luck in separating a coronary peak with a French curve.)

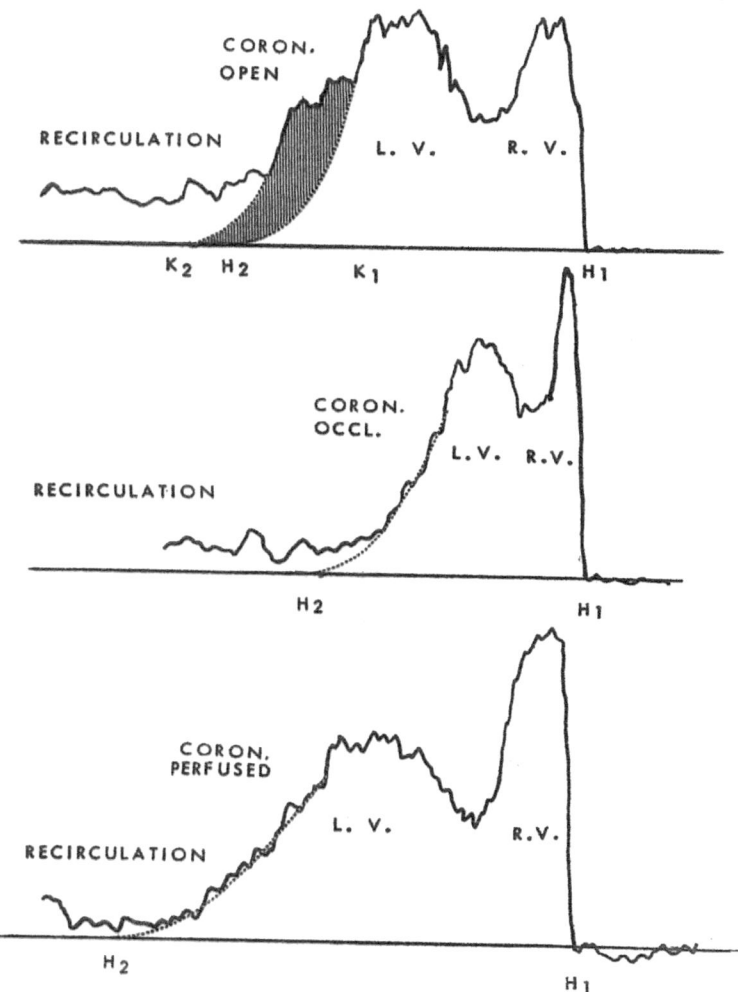

**FIG. 1. Physical Evidence of a Coronary Flow
in the Radiocardiogram.**

My second idea came from playing with a rubber band. If I marked the band close to one end and stretched the band, the band would stretch and the mark would divide the band in two parts with still the same portions of the whole. I tried the idea by injecting an isotope bolus in a plastic tube while water was running through. It was true. The peak concentration of the bolus divided the bolus into two parts that stretched like a rubber band as long as it passed through a tube. This was due to a so-called laminar flow. If, however, the bolus entered a mixing volume, the bolus became dependent on the size of the mixing volume. The relationship of bolus dilution to a volume with different flow dynamics required further exploration.

I contacted the Department for Fluid Dynamics at the University of Oklahoma in Norman, 30 miles south of the city. With the support of the local oil business, the people here were recognized as very knowledgeable. I met with Professor John Powers, Ph.D., and head of the department.

Under Dr. Powers' leadership we did basic *in vitro* work monitoring water flow through plastic tubing and water beakers.

The radiocardiogram represented the amount of tracer over time, provided the monitored volume during its passage through the heart was the same as the volume at the second recording, the recording at the equilibrium state (E). (See Figure 2.) The two recordings had to represent the concentration of tracer in identical volumes. *Additionally, the equilibrium reading (E) represented the radiation in the area after the tracer had been diluted in the total BV. It had to be corrected for this dilution and therefore multiplied by the total blood volume (BV).* This explained why the Huff formula contained a factor for blood volume.

The BV was determined in a well counter from the radiation of the tracer before it was injected into the blood and in a sample of blood at the time of the E-recording. (BV in ml = Concentration/ml before injection divided by the concentration/ml in diluted blood.)

Professor Powers suggested that we set up flow models with different volumes and make a correction factor for each volume. We called the correction factor "Z" and made a chart to mark three points on the washout slope for different volumes. With this Z-factor we could reproduce different washout curves for different volumes and flow rates. (See Figure A-11.)

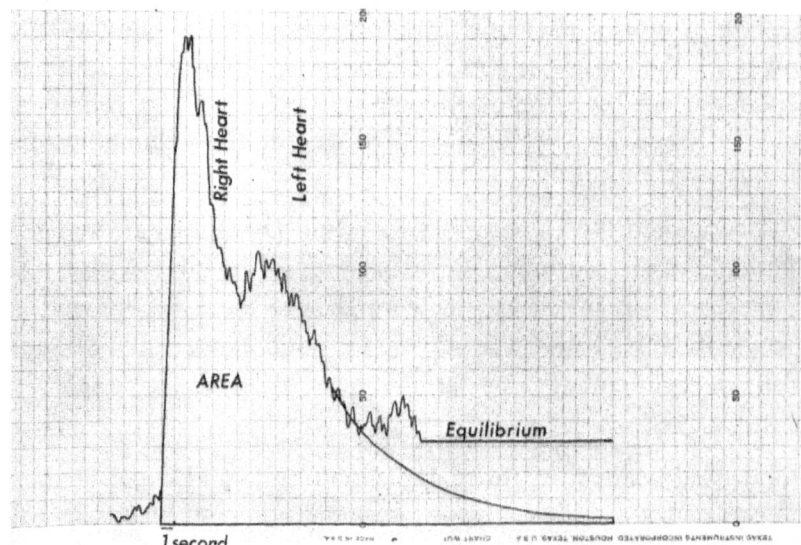

FIG. 2. Normal Radiocardiogram.

For human studies we used two-plane x-ray pictures of the chest, one from the front and one from the left side of the heart, to measure the volume of the heart. Measuring the heart shadow from two directions was recognized to give a good estimate of the total heart volume. Both sides of the heart have the same volume, provided nothing is wrong with the heart valves or there is a shunt between the two sides of the heart. This could be excluded simply by listening to the heart. With help of the Z-curves the radiocardiogram did indeed divide into three flow curves, two for each side of the heart and one for the coronary flow.

The radiocardiogram had now three flow curves but still I could not determine a quantitative coronary blood flow because I had no equation for its calculation.

Brainstorm

Professor Powers went to Germany for one year of sabbatical studies. He sailed with a steamer for relaxation. He wrote me that he had a brainstorm while on the ship and would tell me about it when he returned.

In order to calculate the coronary flow we needed to know how much of the bolus entered into the coronaries and the concentration of the bolus at that time; that is, a time/concentration curve for the coronaries.

From our earlier work with the kidneys we knew that detector sensitivity and geometry of two monitored areas to be compared was important.

The sensitivity could be excluded because we had the same detector for the blood flowing through the coronaries and the heart chambers. The geometries for the scan of the heart as a whole and the coronaries are also the same and are again canceled in the second measurement at the equilibrium (E) state. Scanned volumes from each side of the heart could still be different. Professor Powers used a mean of scanned volumes from each heart side as the total monitored heart volume.

The amount and the concentration of the bolus that went into the coronaries were critical in order to be able to record and calculate flow over time.

A peak of a flow curve represents a time when the amount of the bolus coming into the monitored volume is equal to what leaves the volume. We knew how to separate the radiocardiogram into its three flow curves using the chest x-ray, CO, and the Z-curves. With dividers we could find where the coronary curve was at its tallest; this was the peak of the coronary curve.

The coronary arteries start just outside the left heart at the base of the aorta. There is no diluting volume between the left heart and the coronary arteries. The concentration of the bolus that entered the coronary arteries could be found on the downslope from the left heart at the time below the coronary peak.

The concentration that left the coronaries at that time could be found on the upslope of left heart curve when it had the same concentration. *The area of the left curve represented in the area between these two points* (the striped area in Figure 3) *represented the concentration/time or the flow rate in the coronary arteries.* This was Professor Powers' "brainstorm." The technician received a cookbook recipe with 36 points to follow for the interpretation of the radiocardiogram.

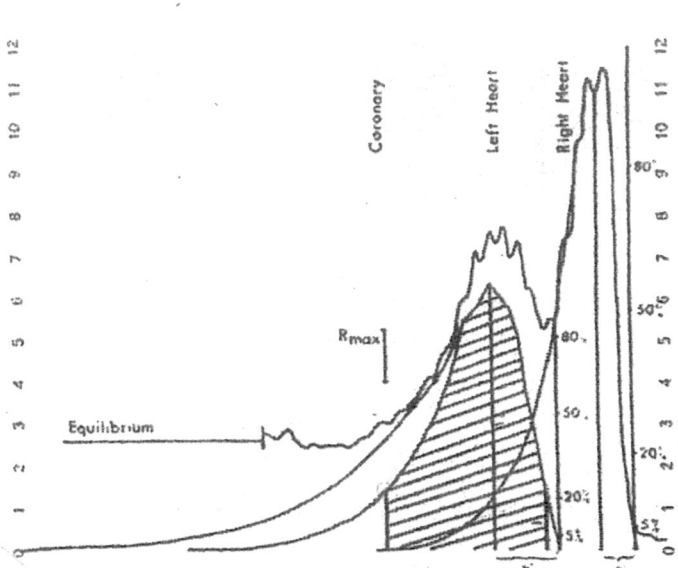

FIG. 3. Radiocardiogram Separated in its Three Main Flow Curves by Scaling and *Z* Factor.

The calculated coronary blood flow, using Professor Powers' formulas yielded a coronary flow of about 4.5 to 5% of the cardiac output, indeed a very reasonable result. The coronary volume from the same curve was 10% of the heart volume, also a very reasonable result according to known information. The coronary flow and coronary volume, the pulmonary volume, and the cardiac output might now be determined from the information in the radiocardiogram. There were also possibilities for looking at shunts, cardiac sac fluids and other important information from the heart and really any abnormality in the circulation. All this information would be available from a single harmless shot in the arm, the radiocardiogram; indeed, a very exciting possibility. Professor Powers described the mathematical derivation in my publication: *Radioisotopes and Circulation*, Little, Brown and Company, 1965. I own the copyrights to this publication and have reprinted pertinent chapters on this subject in the appendices.

Collimator Work

One problem with scanning the peripheral circulation over the heart was to exclude the monitored flows and volumes from any other regions, particularly from the liver. A one-inch thick lead shield surrounded the two-inch crystal in the scintillation detector. The detector crystal had to be retrieved several inches back within the shield so that the detector would have a narrow tunnel vision. This made the whole setup heavy and difficult for the technician to handle.

I designed what I called a "wafer" collimator. The wafer collimator was a half-inch thick lead wafer with 120 1/8-inch small holes or tunnels covering the two-inch front diameter of the crystal. Now the detector could sit next to the skin over the heart without seeing flow or volumes from other organs.

I completed a field identification study that I reported to a medical meeting in New Orleans. The Director from Oakridge National Laboratory was there when I pulled my wafer collimator from my back pocket. He congratulated me for the clever idea and saw also the importance for future scanning with large crystals.

We selected the placement of the detector over the heart with help of a chest x-ray. The collimator limited the field of scanning to that within the heart shadow. There could be some radiation from blood flow in the chest wall. Judging from the experiments with Dr. Snider, this seemed to be very small. A radiocardiogram recorded with these reservations ought to be even more accurate for the determination of cardiac output (CO) than the old-fashioned dye curve because the calibration was automatic in the two recordings, that is, the passage of the bolus and the recording of the steady mixing state, and also because measurements with isotopes are very sensitive and accurate.

St. Louis, 1958
A First Quantitative Verification

Dr. Wolf invited Dr. Richard Bing, Chief of Medicine at the V.A. Hospital at the University of St. Louis to visit us in Oklahoma City. Doctors Wolf and Bing agreed to have me come to St. Louis for one month to compare my technique with another new isotope technique introduced by Dr. Bing. Dr. Bing's technique was based on the Fick principle with a clearance of the positron-emitting isotope Rubidium-84 from the heart muscle. Dr. Bing's technique shows areas of dead heart muscle after a heart attack.

I went to St. Louis in January to compare the two techniques. Dr. Bing assigned Dr. John Danforth to assist me.

John's and my work went very smoothly despite the enormity of machinery that had to be coordinated and work at the same time. We did some ten different measurements. Our flow results followed each other in a 45-degree plot that went through zero.

Miami, 1960
A First Clinical Demonstration

Dr. Johnson arranged for me to examine the therapeutic effect of a vasodilator called Persantine. The pharmaceutical company, Warner Chilcott had had difficulties proving the efficacy of Persantine.

The representative from Warner Chilcott Pharmaceutical came to my laboratory. Dr. Johnson gave a volunteer a tablet and I recorded an obvious dilatation. The factory representative could see the effect on the curve for himself.

Dr. Johnson arranged for Warner Chilcott to sponsor his whole laboratory with six technicians and me to demonstrate the technique at the Annual Meeting of the American Medical Association. To start with, I would stay behind in Oklahoma City to make a movie to illustrate the technique while the technicians and Dr. Johnson sat up the exhibit. The meeting took place in Miami at the huge Miami Convention Center.

Dr. Johnson rented a large booth for the exhibit, had pamphlets printed whereon he was the first name, and also arranged for a TV interview with the Calloway Morning TV show. The arrangements were all done without informing me. The technicians called back to me and told me what was happening.

I soon found out that Dr. Johnson had a personal agenda. There would be thousands of doctors attending. Dr. Johnson had already drawn notoriety for our work and had been given a job as Director for the Radioisotope Laboratory at the Baylor Medical Center in Houston. The new Johnson Space Center was being built here. Dr. Johnson would participate with studies in space medicine.

To be the first name on a scientific report often means that you are the originator. Dr. Johnson, as chief of the laboratory, had always been the second name on any of my reports. I had Dr. Johnson's pamphlets thrown into the Miami canal and new ones printed with mine as the first name. This experience made me suspicious and protective in my future work.

The technicians measured the cardiac output and the coronary flow on any doctor passing by. Hundreds had their heart flow measured. The exhibit got First Prize as the best scientific accomplishment that year.

When I originally started to work under Dr. Johnson, the chief technician in the isotope laboratory Dan Patrick and a college student Sidney Logsdon, were assigned to me. Together, we did much of the modeling with water, plastic tubing and beakers. When we started clinical work, Elaine Patrick, Dan's wife, became the person who read all the curves using the Z-curves, dividers and a planimeter. Elaine worked for me during both the FAA and the Neurocardiology time.

Elaine gave consistency to the interpretation of all the curves and followed a step-by-step recipe when she read the curves. She was very efficient and relieved me from much routine work. Actually, all the technicians were very supportive while I worked in the radioisotope laboratory at the V.A. Hospital in Oklahoma City. My thanks go out to each and every one.

Washington, DC, 1963
A Second Quantitative Verification

When the prediction results began to come in from the long-term studies in the Neurocardiology Center, both Professor Wolf and I began to understand that we had a "tiger by the tail". We had already done one verification study, but it was with another new technique. Professor Wolf suggested and arranged for me to visit the laboratories of Dr. Donald Gregg at the Walter Reed Army Hospital Center in Silver Spring, Maryland outside of Washington, DC. Dr. Gregg's way of measuring coronary blood flow was with electromagnetic flow meters, an undisputedly correct way of determining blood flow through a specific blood vessel.. My absence for a year would not interrupt the research with the scanning of the volunteers.

Dr. Gregg was the recognized world expert on coronary blood flow and had written a book designated to just coronary blood flow.

An electromagnetic flow meter is a magnet that surrounds the artery and creates an electric current from the electrically charged ions in the blood passing through. The current represents the blood flow after the magnet has been calibrated with the same blood. The magnets were placed on vessels of anaesthetized medium to large sized dogs. Dr. Gregg had an expert technician who would build the flow meters by hand. We had to thread the flow meters across the vessel and lock it in place with a small plastic insert-key to close the loop around the vessel.

I reported in to Dr. Gregg. He showed me his lab. A sergeant was assigned to assist me in surgery. We were at least four or five doctors working on different projects.

Dr. Gregg sat down with me and discussed a research plan. Because I was measuring total coronary blood flow, I had first to determine the blood flow in each of the three, (right, left, and septal) coronary arteries. I had to prove that the flow in all of them stayed constant between them during different flow rates. After that, I could compare the sum of the flow rate in the left and right artery with that measured with the isotope. The flow rates had to be determined as percent of the total aortic flow. The aortic flow would be determined with a flow meter placed around the root of the aorta right outside the left heart. Much of this had never been done before. I was surprised that the relative flow rate in the individual arteries was not known. Most studies on the coronaries had been limited to the large main left artery.

This was open heart surgery. I would finally do in medicine what I had originally dreamed of doing—surgery. I was eager to learn and started with watching and helping the other investigators. Similar surgery was done in all rooms, all week long. Everybody had a routine.

Pretty soon I felt ready to start. My first step was to determine the flow in the right coronary as percent of the aortic flow. To dissect the aorta and the right coronary even while the heart was beating was fairly simple in my hands. We, my sergeant and I, threaded a large flow meter across the aorta and a smaller magnet across the right coronary. To record a zero flow for a baseline we used a clamp for the aorta and a snare placed around the right coronary proximal to its flow meter. We used an ephedrine drip to vary the flow rate. After surgery we collected the blood from the dog and calibrated each flow meter we had used. The flow rate in the right coronary remained steady at 15% of the aortic flow through different flow rates.

Next, I had to determine the flow rate in the main left coronary and its septal branch. The septal artery in a 70-pound dog is about 1 mm in diameter, the left artery about 4 mm and the aorta about 15 mm. The septal artery branches off from the underside of the main left coronary vessel about two millimeters from the root of the left artery as it branches off from the aortic root. The septal artery is very short and enters almost immediately into the wall between the two chambers. This makes it crowded at the root of the left coronary. The dissection of the root of the left coronary and placing a small flow meter around it while the heart was beating became a challenge. If the septal artery started to bleed, it was all over. Dr. Gregg designed a genius contraption we likened to a spider because it had so many legs for connections to record flows and pressures.

Zero flow of the aorta was recorded with a clamp. The left coronary was separately perfused from the left carotid artery and the left coronary zero with a snare placed proximal to its flow meter. Flow through for the septal was determined with a snare by subtracting the decrease in flow in the main left when the snare for the septal was pulled close. This all required a very complicated hook-up and could not have been done without Dr Gregg's experienced leadership.

The septal flow was found to be steady at 9% of the left coronary flow and both the left and septal flow stayed at a constant percent of different aortic flow rates.

I was now about seven months into the program but had still not used my isotope technique.

I felt ready for a comparison between the two flow techniques. Dr. Gregg asked for it to be done on a conscious dog with three flow meters and three snares (for right coronary + left coronary + aorta.) My first reaction was that dogs could not survive all the hardware. Dr. Gregg assured that the dogs could survive and insisted it had to be done in a conscious dog.

The flow meters would have connectors and snares pulled through and attached to the skin on the back of the dog. At the start I lost a couple of dogs after such complicated surgery but not many. The dogs would wake up from the anesthesia after about two hours, usually stand up and look pretty cheerful. It was amazing to see. They had to heal for a couple of days before we could do the actual comparison of the two measurements. We would do the surgery on Friday morning. My visiting mother from Sweden and I would come in and care for the dogs on Saturday and Sunday.

Monday I would set up the recording machinery for the electromagnetic flow meters and also for the scanner with its recorder for the radiocardiogram. I used my dog collimator that I had designed for the work with Dr. Snider. We had an intravenous drip going for the injection of the tracer and the medications to vary the flow with. Afterwards, we sacrificed the dogs to calibrate the flow meters. I would inject the isotope and control the two recorders. Two doctors would help with the snares for baselines. It was an elaborate setup.

The whole building was told to be quiet while we did the measurements because the slightest sound would catch the dogs' attention and change the blood flow. It was amazing to see how dynamic blood flow is. The flow in all flow meters would change if the dog lifted its head.

Dr. Gregg thought we needed about 12 different measurements in seven conscious dogs. The flow measurements from the isotope and through the flow meters followed each other within 10%.

First, I needed to write a report on the results from the individual coronary arteries with flow meters. I needed to report that all individual coronary artery flow rate was a constant percent of the aortic cardiac output even when this was changed with epinephrine.

Together with Dr. Gregg, I submitted the report from the septal flow measurements to the *Journal of Applied Physiology*. The report was rejected because we measured the septal flow by occluding it and determined the flow by subtracting it from the total of the left coronary flow.

With this report not accepted, I gave up reporting on the whole subject. I could have spent my life doing this. It was not my calling. The most important for me was that I could trust my clinical tool to assess aging, fatigue, and the risk for heart attack.

Gunnar Sevelius, MD

PART II
Feelings, Fatigue, Aging and Prediction
of a Heart Attack

Federal Aviation Agency (FAA), 1961-1963

The FAA received a large grant to build a research institute in Oklahoma City. FAA was interested in pilot fatigue and pilot aging, both critical for pilot performance.

Dr. Bruno Balke from the new institute asked me if I would be interested in working for him. I explained that I would be, but being on a student visa, I was not eligible for federal employment.

The FAA would take care of my immigration. I would be considered an important scientist. I would be an immigrant on a special quota, signed by the Secretary of State. Secretary Dulles signed the immigration papers for Hilli and I.

Dr. Bruno Balke's first goal was to develop a treadmill test to evaluate pilots' general vascular fitness. A graduated workload on the treadmill would tell about person's vascular fitness or heart muscle reserve. I measured the CO. For this I had to design a portable detector that could be carried on the front of the chest while a person worked on the treadmill. The Tracer Lab Company helped me with a prototype. One could record two measurements, one at rest and one at maximum workload. Coronary flow was difficult to separate because the area of the curve at high workload was too small. Max flow rate at maximum workload could be three times that at rest, an incredible efficiency of the heart muscle.

In order to study fatigue and aging, I had to develop normal values for cardiac output for different ages in males and females.

Normal values of cardiac output were by tradition expressed in a Cardiac Index (CI). Cardiac Index was normalized only for body size and sex, but not for age and not for pulse rate. That CO changed with age had been recognized but was never clinically corrected for. In Figure F-4 is plotted the average cardiac output in different age groups from different investigators together with a regression of

21

cardiac output and age using Dr. Ed Brandt's formula (see Figure 4 below). A 65-year-old man would have half the heart flow of that of a 20 year old.

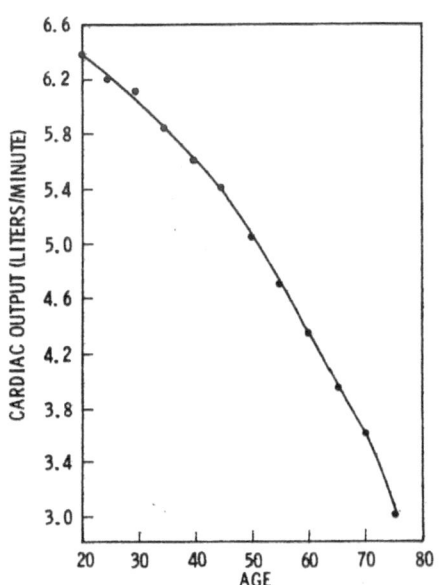

FIG. 4. Age Versus Cardiac Output.

Nurses and laboratory personnel volunteered as females. Veterans, who were discharged for problems other than circulatory, contributed male normal results. The results were submitted for the statistical analysis.

Dr. Edward Brandt, later in his career recognized as U.S. Surgeon General, was the director of the Statistical Department. Ed and his colleagues used some ten different variables and used multi-regression to arrive at two formulas, one for each sex. None deviated from the determined value with more than 10%.

All measurements were done with the patient in resting, supine position without any sedation. The bolus was rushed into the heart by lifting the arm immediately after the injection of the tracer into the antecubital vein.

Cardiac Index or CI is calculated by dividing a factor from the patient's height, weight, and a correction factor called the patient's skin surface area, all with very little relationship with a cardiac output and indeed totally confusing for clinical evaluation. As the plot in Figures 5 and 6 show, the plot of CO versus surface area is almost vertical while the correlation with Ed Brandt's formula (see below) shows a straight distribution line going through zero of the X and the Y-axes.

The clinical evaluation with Ed Brandt's formula is best communicated in percent of the estimated value because some estimated normal values would seem unnecessarily high if the pulse rate and blood volume are high.

Our working hypothesis was that a large blood volume combined with a high pulse rate or small stroke volume would be an early sign of heart muscle fatigue and risk for a blood clot, stroke, or heart attack forming anywhere in the circulation because of the slowing of the blood stream.

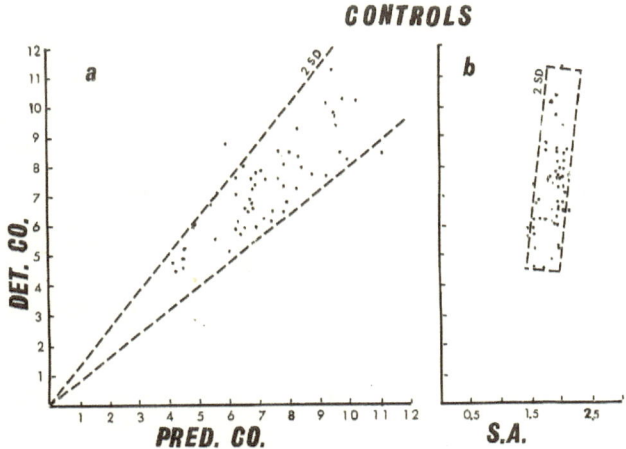

CONTROLS

FIG. 5. Det. CO in Normals vs. Estimated According to Brandt's Formula (a) and vs. Surface Area (b).

We assessed the patients determined cardiac output in two ways: one using patients' pulse rate and measured blood volume at the time of the recording. We called this assessment a

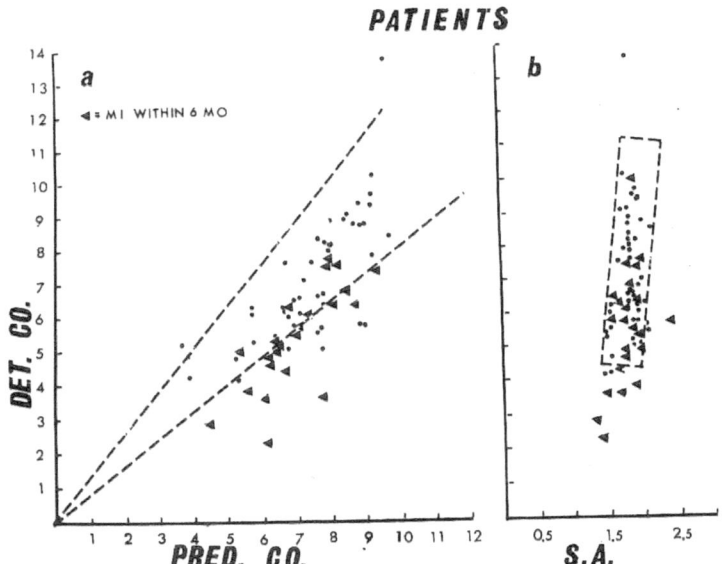

FIG. 6. Repeat of Fig. 5 for Patients. Many of the Values in (b) Fall within 2 SD of Normal Distribution.

hemodynamic assessment. We had a second assessment using a set average of 70 pulse rate and an estimated normal blood volume according to Nadler and Hidalgo Tables 2 and 3. We called this assessment a *metabolic assessment.* We used the hemodynamic assessment in the Prognostic Index (see followup below).

Dr Brandt's two multi-regression formulas for the cardiac output (CO) of normal males and females are listed below. As in all normal distributions the normal ranges are from +20% to –20% of the estimated values.

Males: CO = pulse per minute x 0.0607 +BV (Lit) x 1.67778 – age x 0.05686 – 2.476

Females: CO = pulse per minute x 0.0607 + BV (Lit) x 1.67778 – age x 0.02843 – 2.470

I now had a formula to study aging and fatigue. I could simply compare a determined value with that estimated from Ed Brandt's normal values. The resting heart flow decreased 1% per year from aging in males and slightly slower in females. I confirmed the formulas in men, women and children from two years old to 97 years old. The 97 year old was my neighbor in Oklahoma City. I measured CO on myself and on my mother when she was visiting for her 80th birthday.

The percent difference between a measured and a normalized value of CO corrected for pulse, size, BV, age, and sex hopefully yielded an assessment of the physiological age if permanent, and expressed fatigue if temporary. Hopefully CO and coronary blood flow would indicate what we were looking for—aging and/or fatigue with risk for heart attack.

I stayed with the FAA for two years, assisting Dr. Balke to develop the standardized treadmill test and measuring cardiac output at different workloads.

The Neurocardiology Center, 1963-1969
Flows and Feelings—Risk Assessment
for Heart Attack

Dr. Wolf's lifetime ambition was to study psychosomatic medicine or a connection between emotional feelings and somatic diseases. He applied for and received a very large research grant to organize what became known as the Neurocardiology Center. Eighteen professors and investigators from the Medical Center became engaged within their respective specialties along with 140 volunteers, 70 with history of coronary disease and 70 without such history but matched for sex and age. Most of the volunteers were from a local factory of the General Electric Company. The volunteers were interviewed and examined one to three times a year for the next seven years.

My assignment was to record the radiocardiogram at each visit and also before and during a stress interview by Dr. Wolf. From the radiocardiogram were computed CO, the blood and pulmonary volumes and the coronary flow. All results from the cardiographs were normalized as percent deviation from estimated normal hemodynamic values.

We knew that the heart is a muscle that has to rest between each beat, more effectively so when we rest lying down horizontally and most efficiently when we sleep. At the time of the volunteer visit to the clinic, a research investigator made notes about the volunteers' feelings and life events. At the end of each year we would correlate laboratory tests with the independent clinical notes.

Every year each investigator had to turn in a list of which volunteers were most apt to have a heart attack or vascular incident during the following year. Only Professor Wolf had access to this list of predictions. Once a year we would give a report and Professor Wolf would tell us how we had fared through the year.

When I first compared the patients as a group with their matched controls, I found the patients as a group had a significantly lower cardiac output (p<0.001) and coronary blood flow (p<0.001), but not a significant larger heart volume or BV. Following a one-year observation, I noticed that patients who developed a second heart attack had larger heart volume and BV, with a decrease in their cardiac output and coronary blood flow. To start with, we constructed a Prognostic Index (PI). The PI was based on percent decrease in CO (<1SD=90%) and CBF (<1SD=83%) and percent increase in blood (>1SD=110%) and pulmonary volumes (>1SD=110%). The working theory was that a high PI would be an indication of a fatigued heart muscle.

The total BV is turned over three to four times a minute. All blood vessels are indeed intimately connected in their work of holding the body metabolism at a steady state. The final conclusion was that we needed only the determination of cardiac output and blood volume with a simple radiocardiogram to make the valuable clinical assessment of a person's risk for heart attack and probably also other stroke-like incidences because of the accompanied slowing of the blood stream. This needs to be verified in a very large population over a long period of time. A study group like the one in Framingham would be ideal for verification.

In my final review, I reported how I could actually follow the conditions for heart attack development and, in some situations, predict month by month the precipitation of a stroke or death. Appendix F describes 17 patients with heart attacks, some fatal, with comments from their physicians. There is a striking correlation of low CO with depression and stress/fatigue. The value of a time specific prediction is that most situations are treatable.

The results from the Neurocardiology Center had 7% false negative and 68% true positive results for a specific six-month prediction period, while seeing the patients only routinely once or twice a year.

I made a first report, *Short-term Prediction of Myocardial Infarction or Sudden Death by Hemodynamic Assessment* to a Medical Meeting in Philadelphia in 1975. The host was Dr. M.N. Croll. Eventually Dr. Croll, with three colleagues, L.W. Brady, H.R. Tatem, and T. Honda, published the meeting under the title, *Clinical Dynamic Function Studies with Radionuclides.* I received permission to publish the article from the present copyright owner, McGraw-Hill (see Appendix F).

Dr. Wolf announced that he was moving to the Marine Biological Research Center in Galveston, Texas. The leadership of the support team was shattered.

Below I will quote from the talk I gave for Professor Wolf at his farewell gathering. I called the talk "Flows and Feelings." I started the talk by quoting the German poet, Hermann Neuman, who lived between 1808 and 1875.

Two chambers hath the heart,
There dwelling, live Joy and Pain apart.

The experience that our heart takes part in our feelings is obviously not new in our culture. It shows in our language, in expressions like "warmhearted" and "downhearted." Cupid aims his arrows at the heart and numerous are the poets' lines about the heart housing our feelings.

Figure 7 shows the Prognostic Index (PI) for one of the control patients. The PI is plotted over time in the left column. In the right column are excerpts from the progress notes from the patient's own physician. These were, of course, not available at the time the radiocardiograms were obtained, neither were my results available to the physician at the time the clinician interviewed the patient.

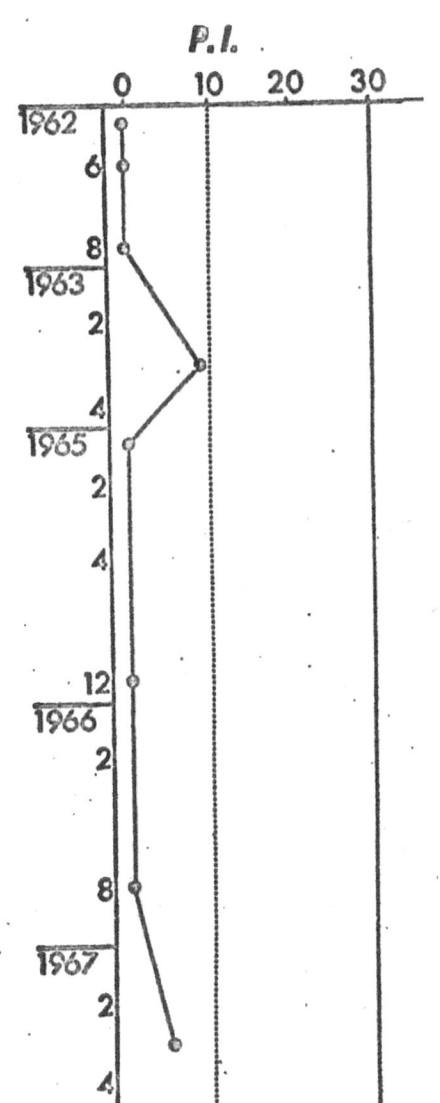

P.I.

| | 0 | 10 | 20 | 30 |

Progress Notes

5/62 Some back pain, nothing new.

6/62 Back and stomach pain, Rx belladonna.

8/62 No complaints today, Rx Donnatal for stomach.

3/63 Tense over business, wife ill with hypertension and MI.

1/65 Wife gone for two weeks, had a good rest after tiresome holidays.

12/65 Slight increase in seasonal workload; otherwise no change, feeling fine.

8/66 Feeling blue, some frustration, early waking; otherwise no change.

3/67 Worked hard last couple of weeks; tired.

FIG. 7. Effect of Stress in a Control Subject.

28

In this control patient you can see his PI stayed at 0, which means that all hemodynamic criteria stayed within 1 SD, with one exception—at the visit in 1963. The progress note in 1963 read "Tense over business being slack; wife back from Mayo Clinic with diagnosis of myocardial infarction and hypertension."

If you follow cardiac output through the record it only varies a few percent from its predicted value. One-third of the subjects in the Neurocardiology Study have even records like this and most of these are from controls. Not only in this measurement, but also in the numerous physiological parameters, did it become evident, and was later statistically proven, that variability in itself is a sign of poor prognosis. (See Figure 8.)

Figure 8 shows the PI from a patient who later died of a myocardial infarction. As he joined the study he started his own business. The business went very slowly for him. He responded by working hard and traveling continuously. He felt depressed and tired but stated, "If I have to, I am going to die with my boots on."

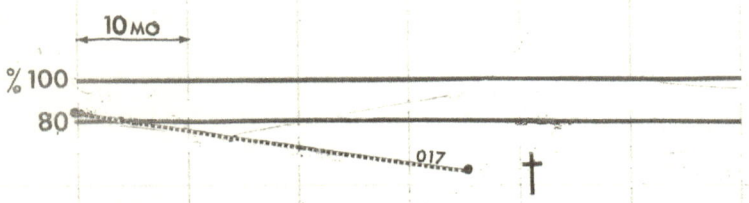

**FIG. 8. Effect of Heavy Workload and Depression
in a Patient Subject.**

Following the PI chart it seems as if he was doing just that. The PI index increases steadily and if one extends this slope it would reach 30 or 3 Standard Deviations around August 1964, the time he actually had his final myocardial infarction. We have not recorded a PI value higher than 30 without the patient being in serious trouble.

Many of the false positive values are from patients with high PI values, and they did not have their infarct within our stipulated time limit of six months but had it later. In clinical work such information would still be very important for corrective measures.

Figure 9 shows the PI values of a retired businessman. He retires and invests his life savings in his old firm. The return from his investments is not as he expected. When he joins the study he is worried. The PI is below two standard deviations. He has a myocardial infarction one month later. Through the seven years in the study he has two more episodes of manifested myocardial infarctions and one hospitalization with severe angina. The first two hospitalizations followed business problems and the last one with his divorce pending; again each occasion proceeded by a peak in the PI chart below two standard deviations.

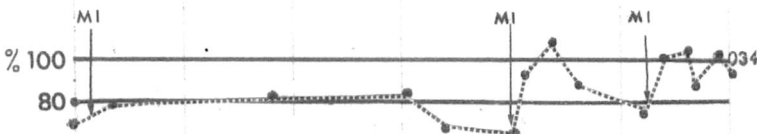

FIG. 9. Effect of Great Variability in a Patient Subject.

Looking back over the record of this retired businessman, who cannot keep his mind off his old business, one may quote Martin Luther:

> *"The human heart is like a millstone in a mill: when you put*
> *wheat under it, it turns and grinds and bruises the wheat to*
> *flour; if you put no wheat, it still grinds on, but then 'tis itself*
> *it grinds and wears away."*

We have ample proof for that worrying and particularly depression influence the flow dynamics of the heart. (See Appendix F.) In the neurocardiology program, eight out of ten myocardial infarctions and eight out of nine deaths due to a circulatory accident were preceded for a six months by a period of depression together with a peak in the prognostic index greater than 2SD. This intimate connection between heart and feelings has been recognized by laymen since ancient times and is most beautifully expressed in Shakespeare's language in *The Winter's Tale*, his last major poem before his death:

Jog on, jog on, the foot-path way
And merrily hent the style:
A merry heart goes all the day,
Your sad tires in a mile.

In this study of the pathophysiology of coronary disease we learned several new medical concepts, such as the hemodynamic efficiency of the heart as a muscle is dependent of both physical and mental rest. Surprising to us was that we had not proposed anything new to the human experience. It comes to show, when we study a disease that has plagued humanity since the earliest of time, we should not hoist our modern knowledge without listening to what history has already learned.

The purpose of the Neurocardiology Center was to predict myocardial infarction within a given timeframe. From the long-term hemodynamic studies much more can be learned. Had the patient's physician specifically known what went on in the patient's heart at the time of the scheduled visit, many of the true positive predictions would have led to specific treatment and a heart attack could have been avoided. If depression or fatigue would have been a specific symptom indicator for the visit, the incidence results might have been even more improved.

A Second Review of the Results

The studies within the neurocardiology program continued. I examined which factor in the PI was the strongest, the CO, CBF, PV or the BV. The CO and blood volume as part of the radiocardiogram procedure proved to be by far the most important factors. The CO determined by the radiocardiogram alone was as effective a predictor as the PI. This could probably have been predicted from the dog experiments in Dr. Gregg's laboratory. The coronary flow was always a given percent of the cardiac output. Having spent 13 years isolating and calculating quantitative coronary flow, I was now faced with the fact that I did not need it for our original goal—the prediction of a myocardial infarction. A simple cardiac output and blood volume determination from a radiocardiogram procedure would be the earliest and almost certainly the best indicator of the risk of a heart attack and probably also for any stroke-like condition.

That was quite a revelation and a main reason for this follow-up publication.

The determination of CO from a radiocardiogram is a very simple procedure. It can eventually be automated, thereby potentially be a very practical clinical test. This is the logical conclusion to draw from the fact that the heart is a muscle that works hard all the time but has also its limits from fatigue and/or depression.

A very sensitive issue still remained. All previous clinical diagnostic studies of CO were normalized according to body size, in the so-called Cardiac Index (CI). I had normalized the CO according to the BV, pulse and age, all according to Ed Brandt's multi-regression formula.

A Cardiac Index cannot identify the few percent changes expressed in a fatigued or aged heart muscle. The CI has statistically a much too wide normal range.

Cardiac pumping at rest is the most fundamental function in body metabolism. All other body functions are dependent on the resting CO. While we perceive ourselves as resting, the heart still works very hard pumping more than a gallon, or 5-6 liters, of blood every minute, turning over the fastest circulatory circuit, that of the coronary, three times a minute and the rest of the circulation almost as fast.

The heart's fatigued-resistance against a temporary demand or an extended high demand is dependent on the physical strength of the heart muscle. The heart muscle in turn is dependent on the blood supply through the coronary arteries.

The coronary flow can certainly be compromised by atherosclerotic buildup blocking the flow that will decrease CO and the fatigue resistance of the heart muscle. On the other hand, a buildup of atherosclerotic plaque does not matter much if the oxygen demand has also decreased with age.

Another factor influencing coronary artery flow is Poiseuille's Law of laminar flow. The flow going through the artery is dependent on the fourth power of the remaining unobstructed diameter. This

Poiseuille effect is easily experienced when one turns off the water of a bathroom faucet. It is only the last turns that close the flow. A 50% occlusion as seen from coronary catheterization may or may not be a critical occlusion. The occlusion needs to be weighted against the size of CO corrected for age and the size of the blood volume; in other words, his or her overall circulatory efficiency. Besides the physical effect of rheology one has to remember that blood in the coronary vessels is really uniquely sucked in and squeezed through the heart muscle as the muscle contracts.

Circulatory efficiency seems to be more dependent on an optimal balance of volumes between the central and the peripheral circulation than on a specific regional flow rate. The quantitative measurement of CO and BV replacing present techniques of trial and error medication in cardiology would most likely be a great improvement in present practices. Further experiences would also lead to more focused treatment.

A circulatory overload syndrome may happen, either from the failing strength of the heart muscle or the failure of the oxygenation of the blood in the lungs, or, of course, from both acting together causing a too large BV for the heart to pump. This led to my trying phlebotomy in three volunteers from the V.A. Hospital. (See Part III.)

Gunnar Sevelius, MD

PART III
Phlebotomy, a Time-Tested
Medical Treatment

Oklahoma City V.A. Hospital, 1966

I have always had an interest in history (see my other recent publications, specifically, *The Nine Pillars of History, an Anthropological Review of 200,000 Years of History, Five Religions, Sexuality and Modern Economics*). A historically common medical treatment in the old times was phlebotomy or "bloodletting." Phlebotomy was such a popular treatment that it was done without any specific diagnosis—often by barbers! So many felt better after phlebotomy that people did not care why.

I had found that the pumping efficiency of the heart was connected to the size of the BV. It made sense that a pump's efficiency should be related to the volume it had to pump.

I proposed a pilot study entitled *The Optimal Relationship Between the Oxygen Carrying Blood Volume, Heart Size and Cardiac* Output. Paraphrasing the text from the proposal:

Working Hypothesis:

Starling's law of the heart states that the heart muscles stretching in diastole force the heart to be stronger in systole. In clinical medicine, this law has been interpreted as an enlargement of the heart is an effective adjustment in response to a damaged heart muscle, such as from an earlier heart attack.

A cited figure from every physiology book, Figure 11 is from work done in 1914. The data are originally from an isolated frog heart. The curve shows that for a diastolic filling up to 20 ml there is a fast increase in systolic power. The systolic contractility increase is lees sharp above 20 ml. Beyond 30 ml of diastolic filling there is a decrease in the contractile force.

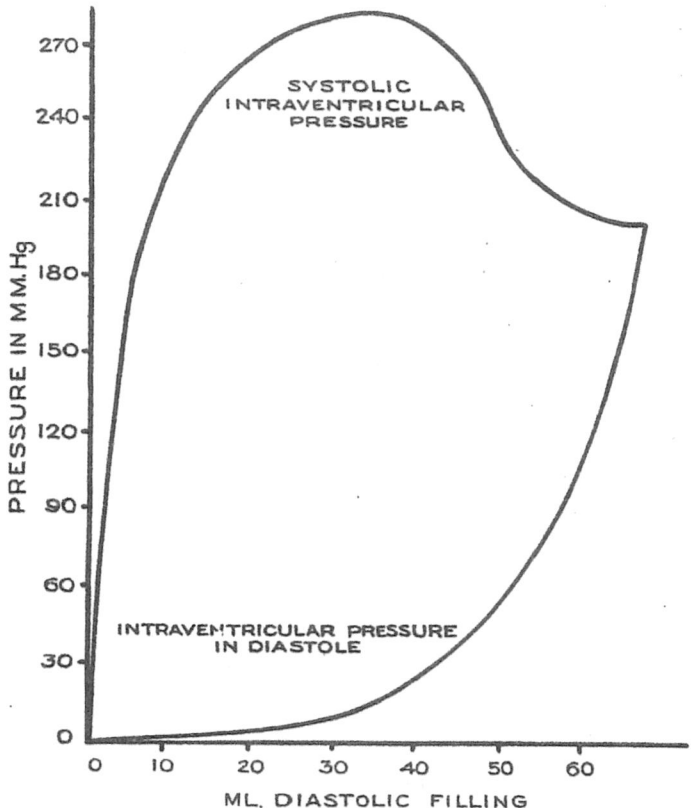

FIG. 11. Influence of diastolic filling upon force of ventricular contraction as shown by systolic intraventricular pressure (upper curve) and diastolic pressure within the ventricle. After the elastic limits of ventricle are reached at about 30 ml, contractions begin to weaken until finally the two curves meet, when systole is incapable of adding to pressure within the ventricle (copied from diagram representing measurements on frog and relabeled to indicate capacity of left ventricle in relation to its systolic and diastolic pressure in a healthy dog's heart weighing 70 grams. By Patterson, Piper and Starling, *J. Physiol.*, 1914, 48:465-513.)

If the stretch of the heart muscle would be an economical solution to an increase in output power it would be likely that the heart would use this *in vivo*. This has never been observed.

For bigger venous return the heart always responds by increasing the pulse rate, never by increasing its stroke volume.

The investigator has measured the heart and BV in 200 people, some with a healthy heart and some with heart failure from coronary insufficiency.

The results from these measurements reveal that even if the BV is normal or enlarged it will distribute itself so that 9 to 10% of it will be inside the heart.

Different things may stimulate an increase in BV. Normally physical activity is a good stimulus. Athletes may have a 20% increase in BV accompanied by bigger heart volume with a larger stroke volume and a resting slow pulse rate. The heart can simply deliver the needed oxygen for body metabolism with fewer beats. The bigger heart volume in athletes is accompanied with an increased mass of heart muscle.

On the other hand, a weak heart muscle may allow fluid in the body to accumulate and may even put the body at a slight oxygen deficit, both leading to an enlarged blood volume. The enlarged blood volume in these patients dilates the inside heart volume because the BV distribution remains with 9% of BV within the heart. This time the heart muscle becomes weaker, with less power per square inch from the inside of heart muscle surface.

An enlarged heart from fluid retention has less fatigue resistance against life's stresses. The now further weak heart muscle leads to further increase in BV, either by retaining fluid or by red cell stimulation, or usually by both. The heart is again further dilated and is getting weaker with decreased CO, all in a continuous circle, eventually leading to a blood clot somewhere in the body.

Doctors try to break this failing circle by giving medicines to stimulate the excretion of the accumulated fluid in the BV and the rest of the body with diuretics without really knowing much about the actual changes taking place in the circulation.

But the oxygen deficit stimulates also the buildup of the red cell part of the BV. Diuretic cannot correct this BV enlargement. Here, I come to the center of my working hypothesis: *This late state of circulatory deficiency needs to be corrected with phlebotomy.*

The investigator argues that this new interpretation of the Starling's law can only be drawn if one measures heart and blood volumes together with CO. It has not been practical to do all these measurements together but the radiocardiogram offers opportunity to do so.

I asked for permission to test the phlebotomy hypothesis in three volunteers at the V.A. hospital. The dates, ID, and results are collected in the tables below.

(1) F.S., a 47-year-old white male with a body surface area of 1.65 m². He had had a previous heart attack. Patient was admitted on 2/22/66 with advanced heart failure. He had been treated with bed rest, digitalis and diuretics until no further improvement could be achieved. He had a first radiocardiogram before he was phlebotomized on 3/2/66. The patient was phlebotomized of 400 ml blood, and the next day another 400 ml. He had a second radiocardiogram on 3/4/66. The results before phlebotomy (A) and the results after (B) are grouped together so they are easily compared. The flow efficiency in milliliters (ml) has to be judged from the percent difference (% diff.) between the determined (D) and the normal estimated cardiac output for each determination. One has to realize that the pulse rate as an expression for a small stroke volume and a determined blood volume even if it is enlarged enters the estimated CO values and expresses the heart pump's efficiency, an efficiency relative to the volume the heart has to pump. It might be more rational to call this estimated CO a Hypothetical Estimated CO. (HE). Hematocrit (Hct) is the percent of blood that consists of red blood cells. CO stands for Cardiac Output, BV for Blood Volume, and HV for Heart Volume determined from the chest x-ray.

Results	D (ml/min)	HE (ml/min)	D/HE (%)	Hct (%)
(A) CO	3280	11000	30	
(B) CO	4330	9400	46	
(A) BV	6677	4632	144	46
(B) BV	5321	4177	127	44
(A) HV	995	601	165	
(B) HV	708	479	148	

The patient had a marked improvement in his well being immediately after the phlebotomy and was discharged after a few days of observation.

(2) S.M., a 42-year-old white male admitted on 4/11/66 with a body surface of 1.9 m^2. He was a schizoid schoolteacher with marked cyanosis from markedly catatonic, poor ventilation of his lungs and with heart failure despite no organic circulatory disease. He was treated with bed rest, digitalis, diuretics and oxygen.

With this treatment the patient had a steady downhill course. On the evening of 4/16/66 the ward physician thought he might loose the patient. The physician decided to phlebotomize the patient of 1000 ml of blood at one time. There was an immediate improvement in the patient's condition. The next morning he could walk to the bathroom by himself. The patient was now given daily intravenous drip of Dexapram to stimulate his breathing. The patient started to diurese and the IV infusion was stopped.

The patient had three radiocardiograms (RCG), one before phlebotomy (A), one after phlebotomy (B), and one just before he was discharged (C). We will group all three RCGs together as done in Patient 1, FS. The hematocrit and the venous oxygen saturation (VOS) are again reported in percentage.

RCG	D (ml/min)	HE (ml/min)	D/HE (% diff.)	Hct %	VOS %
(A) CO	6450	12450	52	61	38
(B) CO	11400	14000	81	50	51
(C) CO	9070	9400	96	47	40
BV					
(A) BV	6650	5060	131	61	38
(B) BV	8240	5060	162	50	51
(C) BV	5540	4507	121	47	40
HV					
(A) HV	844	529	141	61	38
(B) HV	973	741	131	50	51
(C) HV	534	490	109	47	40

(3) J.P. was a 41-year-old white male farmer with history of a previous myocardial infarction and now admitted on 3/31/66 for fibrillating heart, and heart failure with an enlarged heart volume. He was treated for one month with complete bed rest, digitalis and "any and all" diuretics on the market. I was given permission to handle the phlebotomy. The patient had seven radiocardiograms. I made the comments in the chart below.

After his last phlebotomy there was no improvement in heart pumping efficiency. Hemoglobin recovered in four days. It is possible the BV before the last phlebotomy is ideal for his fibrillating heart and the patient as well as we can get him. The patient went home over the weekend, had a BBQ dinner and made love to his wife. The patient was discharged the following week.

RCG Date	D (ml/min)	HE (ml/min)	D/HE (% diff.)	Hct %	VOS %	Weight (kg)
Patient on complete bed rest, unable to go to the bathroom.						
4/8 CO	2.8*	14.0	20	57	55	76
4/27 CO	2.68	12.2	22	58	60	72
5/3 CO	500 ml phlebotomy					
5/4 CO	500 ml phlebotomy					
*This CO was the lowest I had so far recorded. I used this CO to estimate maximum life expectancy. People with a heart pumping only 20% of his/her hypothetical normal could still be alive at 120 years of age (+/–2SD or 20%), but certainly not take part in much activity.						
5/5 Patient markedly improved, could get out of bed and go to the bathroom.						
5/5 CO	4.14	12.2	34	50	83	72
5/8 CO	3.24	10.6	31	50	82	63
5/8	250 ml phlebotomy					
5/9	400 ml phlebotomy					
5/10 Patient was up most of the day and clinically much improved. Blood hemoglobin was at first 14 gm but recovered within three days.						
5/10 CO	3.35	9.6	35	45	75	62
5/17 Patient felt better than he had for years. He took his meals in the dining room. His heart was still fibrillating.						
5/17 CO	6.16	10.2	60	45	40	61
5/18	325 ml phlebotomy					
5/19	325 ml phlebotomy					
5/20 CO	5.89	9.6	61	45	55	60

The different blood and heart volumes measured at each RCG date were as follows:

Date	BV		
	D ml	**E ml**	**% Diff.**
4/8	7320	4752	154
4/27	7400	4700	156
5/5	7261	4752	153
5/8	6335	4422	143
5/10	5740	4420	130
5/17	5800	4400	132
5/20	5700	4300	132

Date	HV from Chest X-ray		
	D ml	**E ml**	**% Diff.**
4/8	1111	660	168
4/27	1100	666	165
5/5	840	648	130
5/8	971	570	170
5/10	829	517	160
5/17	800	517	155
5/20	689	517	133

I got busy and did not have time to follow up this short pilot study. Still, I could not disregard it and saved my results. My impression from blood flow rheology is that diuretics, usually the first treatment for heart failure, are effective because they are non-invasive corrections of the BV. They are effective until there is no more free fluid to excrete. At this point, when a large BV remains, phlebotomy is the only effective solution to a condition that eventually will shorten life. One may have to repeat phlebotomy but this is still worthwhile because it is such a simple procedure. This is what the old and wise found out by trial and error. From my own experience in advanced age I think that many decisions in cardiology are still based on trial and error. I believe the RCG has much to give to medical practice but results here need to be confirmed independently. Because of my age I am eager to have the work verified. I may need phlebotomy myself.

PART IV
Health Education and
Heart Attack Prevention

National Aeronautics & Space Administration, 1970
Clinical Applications of the Oklahoma Experiences

With my background from the Neurocardiology Center, I could probably be of most use to society in the area of preventive medicine. Even if not all of my work had been recognized, I knew something unique about the pathophysiology of myocardial infarcts, an important factor for leaders in both industry and government.

The Silicon Valley was already growing very fast. The most respected Palo Alto Medical Clinic had for several years cared for the dispensary of the local NASA station at Moffett Field. The contract was up for renewal. In December 1970 President Nixon signed into law the creation of the OSHA Agency for occupational health and safety. Dr. Joseph LaDou was in the process of setting up an industrial medical clinic in a small building not far from Moffett Field. It was probably one of the first independent medical clinics in the country devoted totally to industrial health. Joe applied for the contract to care for the NASA employees, with me as its local Medical Director. Dr. Stein, the local NASA Medical Administrator, interviewed me. Joe and I won the new contract.

While at NASA, I started to write about health fitness. I wrote one article about how to train for cardiovascular fitness. The training was based on the simple method of intermittently stimulating the heart muscle with high (120) and low (80) pulse rate, and eventually adding the high pulse periods together. Professionals should do this in high altitude. This was how my high school running idol, Gunder Hägg, had come to become the running world champion in the 1940s.

One of the NASA employees recommended me to "Runner's World." The article was rewritten for the up and coming journal,

The Runner, a journal that had its main office locally but subsequently became the national journal for committed runners.

Besides the contract for the regular dispense work at NASA, we received a contract to supervise a study of weightlessness. At the time I did not know, but this was a similar study Dr. Phillip C. Johnson did on weightlessness for NASA in Houston, a *"cute"* coincidence.

I had worked for NASA for two years when the Medical Director for Lockheed Missile and Space Company, Dr. John Preston, called me and said he planned to retire and suggested me as his replacement. I went for an interview and hired in as Lockheed's Medical Director. I was now responsible for the working health of close to 27,000 employees.

Lockheed Missile & Space Corporation, 1972
Health Education in a Large Working Population

Lockheed had a reputation as a *"heart killer."* There had been several layman publications in the local press to this effect. Employees did indeed have a stressful work. They had to apply for new federal contracts on a timely basis in competition with other companies, sometimes getting the contract and sometimes not. Without a contract employees had to look for another job. Besides, when they had worked hard to finish a contract, they again had to go looking for a new job. Fortunately, Lockheed was very large with many job opportunities, but still, such contract work could be very stressful.

The good reception at NASA of my booklet about training for physical fitness inspired me to do a similar booklet about exercise for Lockheed employees. The administration encouraged me to expand the program for other health risk factors. I added booklets on "High Blood Pressure," "Smoking," "Stress Control" and "Weight Control." I also designed a "Stress Control Calendar" that helped employees plan their personal and work schedule.

At the same time, I introduced a computer program so that I could follow lost work time along with its medical reason. The program listed 12 body systems, such as skeletal, skin, respiratory, urinary and ten different kinds of exposure such as trauma, infection, degenerative, etc. The program had some specific identifiers, like heart attack, high blood pressure, and smoker or nonsmoker. By combining body systems with reasons and habits, we could have a continuous idea of the health and health habits in our working population.

This was the time, 1998, when Dr. Donald Abraham was the first to recognize a new disease—AIDS in San Francisco. Society in general was scared that AIDS was contagious. I visited the newly opened AIDS Clinic in San Francisco and met with Dr. Abraham on the new AIDS ward with all the seriously ill, young males. Dr. Abraham explained the pathophysiology and agreed to help me in writing an informative health pamphlet for the Lockheed employees. Our medical clinic thought we knew of one AIDS-infected employee. Dr. Abraham assured me there was no risk of contamination in the workplace. I gave a presentation to top management, and thanks to my computer program, I could assure the management there was no risk for employee contamination. Lockheed was the first major employer to decide not to have any discriminative hiring or workplace rules for employees with AIDS.

I arranged for SRI International of Menlo Park, California, to study the incidence of high blood pressure and the incidence of heart attacks in different departments. The assumption was that working without deadlines in administration or auditing would have lower stress than working under contract deadlines. Doctors Joseph H. Chadwick, Ph.D., Margaret A. Chesney, Ph.D. and Michael Feuerstein, Ph.D. at SRI International were the leaders of the study and totally unassociated from the Lockheed organization.

After several years of followup, the SRI team could report that although stress was high in people working under contract deadlines they, as a group, were high-energy people, physically fit, with fewer incidences of high blood pressure and myocardial infarcts. In general, Lockheed employees were well informed in caring for their bodies, had less incidence of high blood pressure, and fewer heart attacks. The incidence rate of myocardial infarcts at Lockheed was 3% at the start of the study versus 9% in the general population, and decreased to 2% during the 1980-1984 study.

SRI could show that smoking decreased from 22% to 15% in a rather short time, thanks to employee education. The computer program also revealed that smokers had no difference in lost work time as compared to nonsmokers. Damage to the lungs from smoking seemed to cause serious sickness later than in working life. Management still introduced dedicated smoking areas and smoke-free group meetings. Lockheed Corporation also donated part of the ground for the building of an exercise area.

Lockheed set a first world record for mass weight control, losing 14.584 pounds of blubber in six weeks. The campaign was written up for the *Journal of Occupational Medicine*.

We studied different techniques for mass health education. To distribute campaign material to over 100 buildings became a distribution problem. We found that the best way to spread medical information was to have a standing exhibit with booklets in the office of the Credit Union. Here all employees would visit rather frequently. They would pick up booklets on the subjects that concerned themselves or their families *just at the time of personal concern*.

We would also initiate different promotional programs with flyers and posters at certain times of the year. For instance, alcohol or smoking programs before Christmas, weight control after New Year or in the spring, stress control at tax time, and exercise in the summertime. Pretty soon we had health as a major subject of conversation among all the employees and peer pressure effectively assisting us.

The educational programs became popular with management. My booklets and posters were distributed to all divisions of Lockheed, some 100,000 employees. I continued to expand my educational program for employees and added programs on "Back Care and Lifting Techniques," "Hearing Control," "Dental Health," "Family Support" and "You are It—First Aid" for what to do in an emergency, while you wait for help.

We added a booklet on alcohol and drug addiction. With management's blessing, I started an alcohol rehabilitation program and formed a committee of AA members among the employees. One of the committee members was elected and recommended to management to lead a dedicated alcohol program for the total workforce. Eventually this program became independent from the medical department.

The fundamental technique for creating a behavioral change in a large industrial population has two steps: 1) *convenient access* to credible medical information, and 2) *enhanced peer pressure* in seasonal campaigns with posters and flyers.

The health care cost per 1,000 employees was 33% less in the Lockheed plant in Northern California, with intense health promotion versus the plant in Southern California with less intense health education, despite similar age and sex distribution in both plants.

An exhibit about the Lockheed Health Education Program was shown at numerous industrial medical meetings. Local colleges with Health Education Departments recognized internships in the Lockheed Medical Department.

El Camino Hospital was the regional hospital for referrals from our medical department. Lockheed initiated a first computerization of its medical records. Professional journals now recognize El Camino Hospital as the most technically advanced hospital in the world.

One of my most lasting contributions has been to accept Dr. Wesley Alles, with a Ph.D. in health promotion from Pennsylvania State University. Wes elected to work with me during his sabbatical year. He stayed on and took over the management of health promotion at Lockheed. I recommended Wes to lead the Health Improvement Program at Stanford University, and from there he was offered to consult in a national Health Education program for YMCA's office in Chicago. Wes is still leading the Health Education at Stanford and is now also the Chairperson of the Board of El Camino Hospital, the tone setting regional hospital in the Silicon Valley. Wes has become one of my closest friends.

Lockheed gave me the copyrights to its health education program. In retirement, I have now updated and digitized the text of these publications. I have called them *Add Years to Your Life and Life to Your Years, Parts I and II.* They are available through my blog:

http://www.ninepillars.com

http://web.me,com/gsevelius/Site/Home.html

I have now been retired for more than 20 years. This report is largely written from old notes and memory. I have had a happy and challenging life. In retirement I have kept busy thinking back, contemplating over history and my own life, what I did and what I did not have time or a chance to do.

With this, I wish you: "Live Well."

—Gunnar

APPENDIX A
FUNDAMENTALS OF DATA
INTERPRETATION

John E. Powers & Gunnar Sevelius

RADIOACTIVE TRACER TECHNIQUES at present play an important role in clinical studies and diagnosis. The application of surface monitoring of radioactive injections is of increasing importance, and details of techniques which are currently in clinical use will be presented in subsequent chapters. The potential for continued development of clinical techniques based on use of surface monitoring is very great. The additional research required can be aided in many ways by mathematical analysis and experiments with physical models. Therefore, the purpose of this chapter is twofold: (1) to present the fundamentals of data interpretation to serve as a basis for a clearer understanding of the details of various clinical techniques which will be given in later chapters, and (2) to stimulate further research by presenting the mathematical basis for several techniques which appear to have some promise but which have never been tested either experimentally or clinically.

The chapter is arranged in order of increasing equipment requirements for the analysis, and this order also corresponds well to that of increasing mathematical complexity. Thus, much information is obtainable from equilibrium measurements made with a very simple scanner. More information is discernible from the time variation of radioactive injections as obtained by use of a recorder in combination with a scanner. And finally, correct interpretation of simultaneous determinations of two or more time-dependent variables yields additional useful information. Under each of these major topics an attempt will be made to discuss the techniques in a very general manner, apply mathematics to develop the relations necessary for proper interpretations of the data, and describe and discuss applicable experiments with physical models whenever such data are available.

INTERPRETATION OF EQUILIBRIUM ACTIVITY DATA

If a suitable radioactive material is injected into the blood stream, it will soon distribute itself uniformly throughout the entire vascular system. Comparatively simple equipment can be used under such conditions to obtain valuable information relative to volumes.

49

DILUTION STUDIES

It is virtually impossible to make a direct determination of the total volume of blood contained in the vascular system. Instead, a rather simple dilution technique is used.

The radioactive substance to be used in dilution studies (and in other techniques to be discussed in subsequent sections) must be chosen with care. It obviously must be nontoxic; further, it should be sufficiently active for proper analysis but not so active as to be dangerous. The half-life of the isotope should be long enough so that reduction in activity during the course of the experiment does not complicate interpretation of the results. The material should remain in the vascular system during the course of the determination but be eliminated from the body fairly soon thereafter.

After a suitable radioactive material has been selected, the volume, v, and net count rate, R, of a small amount is determined and this material injected into the vascular system. Care is taken to allow for background count rates, as well as for the material that remains in the syringe. After a sufficient time has elapsed, the radioactive material will be uniformly distributed throughout the vascular system and a small sample of blood is then removed. The volume, v', and the count rate, R', of this sample are carefully determined. In addition to giving due consideration to the background count rate it is necessary that the two count rates, R and R', of volumes v and v', respectively, be determined under conditions of identical geometry. The total blood volume, V_t, is then calculated as follows:

$$V_t = v' \frac{R}{R'} - v \qquad (1)$$

Under most conditions the volume, v, will be negligible with respect to the total blood volume, V_t, so that v in general will not even be determined in the course of the experiment.

The mathematical justification of Equation 1 is very straightforward: Care was taken to insure that the net amount of radioactive material that entered the body, I, was determined by monitoring according to the relation

$$R = \alpha I \qquad (2)$$

where α is a geometrical and scanner factor. The radioactive material has distributed itself uniformly by the time a sample is withdrawn and therefore is in uniform concentration, C, throughout:

$$C = \frac{I}{V_t + v} = \frac{I'}{v'} \tag{3}$$

where I' is the total amount of radioactivity contained in the withdrawn volume v'. Note that this relation assumes that the total radioactivity, I, in the combined volumes, $V_t + v$, is equal to the net amount injected. This will only be the case if the decline in radioactivity due to decay is negligible and the amount of radioactive material that leaves the vascular system is very small during the time interval between injection and withdrawal of the sample.

As mentioned previously, the total radioactivity will not be known; instead, monitored amounts R and R' will be determined where

$$R' = \alpha' I' \tag{4}$$

and Equation 2 expresses a similar relation for R. Substitution of Equations 2 and 4 into Equation 3 and solution for V_t yields

$$V_t = v' \frac{\alpha R'}{\alpha' R} - v \tag{5}$$

In general the geometric and instrument factors α and α' will not be known. Use of the same scanner to determine R and R' plus careful attention to geometric factors will insure that α and α', in which case Equation 5 reduces to Equation 1.

PROPORTIONAL SCANNING

In addition to determining total blood volume as described in the preceding paragraphs, it is often desirable to be able to locate individual pools of blood and estimate their volumes. The technique of proportional scanning is applicable.

Consider an experiment in which volumes of different sizes are filled with a solution of radioactive material of uniform concentration. As described in detail above, the radioactive material should remain in solution (i.e., it should neither volatilize into the air nor be absorbed by the surface of the container) and should have a long half-life. The various volumes are arranged so that they are in view of the scanner and are all located in geometrically similar positions relative to the scanner as shown in Figure A-1.

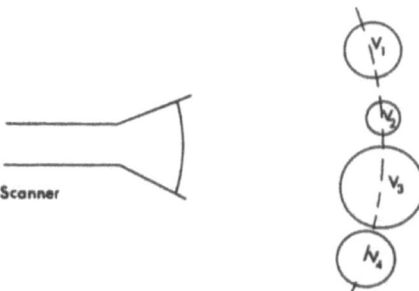

FIG. A-1. Volumes of random size arranged in geometrically similar positions relative to a scanner.

If the net count rate registered by the scanner is R_t when all four volumes are in view and a net reading of R_{t-2} is registered when volume V_2 is either removed or blocked by shielding from the view of the scanner, then volume V_2 is related to the total volume, $V_t = V_1 + V_2 + V_3 + V_4$, by the relation

$$V_2 = V_t \left[1 - \frac{R_{t-2}}{R_t} \right] \qquad (6)$$

The mathematical justification of this relation is similar to that for dilution. It is assumed that the vessels contain material of uniform concentration, C, such that

$$C = \frac{I_t}{V_t} = \frac{R_t}{\alpha_t V_t} = \frac{I_2}{V_2} = \frac{R_2}{\alpha_2 V_2} \qquad (7)$$

where I_t is the total amount of radioactive material contained in all four volumes (V_t) and α_t is the geometrical factor relating R_t to I_t as in Equation 2. Removal of the radioactive material in V_2 from the view of the scanner reduces the scanner reading accordingly.

$$R_{t-} = R_t - R_2 \qquad (8)$$

Division of the three terms in this expression by R_t yields

$$\frac{R_{t-2}}{R_t} = 1 - \frac{R_2}{R_t} \qquad (9)$$

The ratio R_2 / R_t is related to volume by applying Equation 7:

$$\frac{R_2}{R_1} = \frac{\alpha_2 I_2}{\alpha_1 I_1} = \frac{\alpha_2 C_2 V_2}{\alpha_1 c_1 V_1} \tag{10}$$

Under conditions such that $\alpha_2 = \alpha_1$ and the concentration is uniform throughout ($C_2 = C_1$), Equation 10 is combined with Equation 9 to yield

$$\frac{R_{1-2}}{R_1} = 1 - \frac{V_2}{V_1} \tag{11}$$

Solution of this relation for V_2 yields Equation 6.

TRAVERSE SCANNING

In some cases it will not be practical to scan all volumes simultaneously, but it may be possible to scan the volumes individually under conditions of similar geometry and interpret the data in terms of relative volumes.

If this technique is to be applied properly, the individual volumes must contain a suitable radioactive tracer in uniform concentration as described in the preceding section. If equilibrium count rates can be determined on the individual volumes so that geometric similarity is maintained, the volume ratios will be the same as the ratios of equilibrium count rates.

$$\frac{V_1}{V_2} = \frac{R_1}{R_2} \tag{12}$$

where the subscripts 1 and 2 are used to identify individual volumes.

The mathematical justification follows from the relations between the count rate R, the total amount of radioactivity, I, and the concentration, C, as previously discussed.

$$R_1 = \alpha_1 I_1 = \alpha_1 C_1 V_1 \tag{13}$$

$$R_2 = \alpha_2 I_2 = \alpha_2 C_2 V_2 \tag{14}$$

The ratio R_1/R_2 is therefore

$$\frac{R_1}{R_2} = \frac{\alpha_1 C_1 V_1}{\alpha_2 C_2 V_2} \tag{15}$$

Under conditions of uniform concentration $C_1 = C_2$ and if it is possible to so arrange the scanner that $\alpha_1 = \alpha_2$, Equation 15 reduces to Equation 12.

It will in general be quite difficult to arrange a scanner relative to different volumes so that geometric identity is obtained. Another factor of importance in applying Equation 12 should be noted: V_1 and V_2 as included in Equations 13-15 are the volumes which are in view of the scanner. If the volume being scanned is large, it may be that part is excluded from the view of the scanner. If the volume being scanned is small, it is probable that other volumes such as those attributable to connective tubing are included. As a result one would expect that large volumes might appear to be smaller than actual and small ones to be larger than actual.

INTERPRETATION OF TIME-ACTIVITY CURVES

In the preceding discussion it was assumed that sufficient time had passed following injection of radioactive material to allow uniform distribution throughout the entire vascular system. Determinations made under these conditions require relatively simple equipment. Much more information can be obtained when a recorder of some type is used with a ratemeter and the activity following injections is recorded as a function of time. In such determinations the total amount of radioactivity contained in a monitored volume will be recorded by surface monitoring. Several determinations may be made simultaneously and/or the variation of concentration at a point may also be measured and used in conjunction with surface monitoring determinations. The purpose of this section is to consider the proper interpretation of the data so derived. The first part will cover interpretation of data obtained by monitoring with a single scanner, and the second part will consider information yielded by proper interpretation of two or more simultaneous determinations.

USE OF A SINGLE MONITOR-RECORDER

Proper interpretation of time-activity curves obtained with a single scanner and coupled recorder provides valuable information in regard to volumes of individual organs, flow rate through organs, and rate of clearance. These three topics are discussed in the following sections.

VOLUME DETERMINATION BY CLOSED SYSTEM DILUTION. In addition to the proportional and traverse scanning methods for the determination of the volume of individual organs, it is also possible to utilize time-activity determinations to estimate the volume of individual organs. In making such a determination a small amount of a suitable radioactive material is injected directly into the monitored volume as rapidly as possible. It is desirable to make the injection as far from the exit of the organ as possible and as near to the organ's geometric center as possible. In general, a compromise in positioning of the injection will be required. The entire volume should be scanned, but as little else as possible. The monitor should be in a fixed position relative to the organ being scanned. The recorder used should have a rapid response so that the maximum recorded count rate, R_{max}, is attained quickly. The level of radioactivity will decrease from the maximum and will eventually become constant at E, indicating that equilibrium has been reached in the closed system. Under these conditions the monitored volume, V_M, is related to the total volume of the closed system, V_t, by the following equation:

$$V_M = V_t \frac{E}{R_{max}} \qquad (16)$$

The mathematical substantiation of this simple relation is similar to that presented in previous sections. If the injection is rapid and the instrument response is also rapid, the maximum reading, R_{max}, will occur with all of the radioactive material, I, in view of the scanner.

$$R_{max} = \alpha I \qquad (17)$$

The equilibrium reading, E, will occur after the total dose, I, has been uniformly distributed throughout the total volume, V_t.

$$E = \alpha'I' = \alpha'CV_M = \alpha'\frac{I}{V_t}V_M \qquad (18)$$

Combination of Equations 17 and 18 and rearrangement to express the result in terms of V_M yields:

$$V_M = V_t \frac{\alpha E}{\alpha'R_{max}} \qquad (19)$$

If care is taken to inject the tracer near the geometric center of the organ and the position of the scanner relative to the organ is kept constant, the geometric factor at the instant of injection, α, should have the same value as the geometric factor at equilibrium, α', and under these conditions Equation 19 reduces to Equation 16.

Only two values, R_{max} and E, are utilized in the determination; therefore, a complete time-activity curve is not essential to the determination.

FLOW RATE DETERMINATIONS. The determination of flow rates through various organs is perhaps the most important application of time-activity curves obtained from surface monitoring. The convenience, rapidity, and accuracy of this method have been recognized by many, and its application will be expanded in the future. A small volume of a suitable radioactive substance is injected into the stream which enters the monitored volume (rather than into the volume itself), and a continuous record is kept of the activity within the monitored volume. The data provided by this record can be interpreted in several ways, as will be discussed below.

It is desirable to interpret time-activity curves in such a way that a minimum of assumptions is required. The first development presented below calls for very few assumptions and yields an equation that is used in further developments. The equation is referred to as the *basic flow equation*.

In brief, if a suitable radioactive tracer in total amount I enters a stream of volumetric flow rate F that passes through a monitored volume V_M and the area under the time-activity curve A is determined, these factors and the geometric factor α are related as follows:

$$A = \alpha I \frac{V_M}{F} \tag{20}$$

This basic flow equation is justified mathematically by considering that the material flowing through the volume is composed of very small amounts of radioactive material which pass through the volume as a unit. A typical unit has a total count rate δI_n and while in view of the scanner contributes the amount δR_n to the total reading of the scanner.

$$\delta R_n = \alpha_n \delta I_n \tag{21}$$

The length of time the particles remain in the monitored volume differs from particle to particle but is equal to λ_n for this particular particle. This particle contributes to the total area A an amount δA_n given by

$$\delta A_n = \lambda_n \delta R_n = \lambda_n \alpha_n \delta I_n \tag{22}$$

The total area is the summation of the individual areas.

$$A = \Sigma \delta A_n = \Sigma \lambda_n \alpha_n \delta I_n \tag{23}$$

The evaluation of the summation requires a knowledge of the number of particles and the corresponding values of their residence times, λ_n. For our purposes it will be convenient to consider an *average residence time* together with an average geometric factor, α, such that Equation 23 reduces to

$$A = \alpha \lambda_{ave} \Sigma \delta I_n = \alpha \lambda_{ave} I_M \tag{28}$$

where I_M refers to that part of the injected dose that passes through the monitored volume.

The radioactive material is transported through the monitored volume V_M by a fluid whose volumetric flow rate if F_M. Therefore, the average residence time of the transporting fluid, λ'_{ave}, is as follows:

$$\lambda'_{ave} = \frac{V_M}{F_M} \qquad (29)$$

Under most conditions the radioactive material will be well mixed with the transporting material and will therefore have the same flow characteristics, such that

$$\lambda'_{ave} = \lambda'_{ave} = \frac{V_M}{F_M} \qquad (30)$$

The basic flow equation can be developed from a slightly different viewpoint in order to relate the average residence time to a function, $\phi(\lambda)$, that relates the residence time to the number of particles having particular residence times. In particular, if dI_n represents the total count rate of all particles with residence time, λ_n, then the contribution of all such particles to the total area is

$$dA_n = \alpha_n \lambda_n D I_n \qquad (24)$$

The function $\phi(\lambda)$ relates dI_n to the total amount of radioactive material that passes through the monitored volume, I_M, in that the fraction of particles with residence times between λ_n and $\lambda_n + d\lambda$ is given by $\phi(\lambda)d\lambda$. Thus Equation 24 becomes:

$$dA_n = \alpha_n \lambda_n [I_M \phi(\lambda) d\lambda] \qquad (25)$$

Accepting the idea of an average geometric factor as before and integrating to determine the total area yields

$$A = \alpha I_M \int_0^\infty \lambda \phi(\lambda) d\lambda \qquad (26)$$

Comparison of Equations 28 and 26 yields a relation between λ_{ave} and $\phi(\lambda)$

$$\lambda_{ave} = \int_0^\infty \lambda \phi(\lambda) d\lambda \qquad (27)$$

It is rare that the function $\phi(\lambda)$ is known; Equation 27, therefore, is of limited practical value.

Substitution of Equation 30 into Equation 28 yields

$$A = \alpha I_M \frac{V_M}{F_M} \tag{31}$$

One is generally interested in determining the flow rate, F, through an entire organ rather than the flow rate through only the monitored volume, F_M. However, if the isotope is uniformly distributed throughout the stream, the amount of radioactive material in a portion of the stream will be in direct proportion to the amount of flow of that portion.

$$\frac{I_M}{F_M} = \frac{I}{F} \tag{31a}$$

Substitution of Equation 31a into Equation 31 yields the basic flow equation, Equation 20. This development establishes the conditions under which it applies. It should be noted that the basic equation will not apply under conditions such that the radioactive substance is absorbed inside the monitored volume and, as a result, has a much higher residence time than the carrying fluid; it will not apply under conditions of recycle in which case the radioactive material passes through the monitored volume more than once; and it *may* not apply under conditions of maldistribution of tracer in the flowing stream.

The basic flow equation is so important in the determination of flow rates by surface monitoring that several experiments were conducted with apparatus constructed of glassware and tubing to test the validity of the assumptions incorporated in its development. The basic experimental arrangement is shown schematically in Figure A-2.

As Figure A-2 indicates, water flows from a tank in which a constant level of water is maintained, through surgical rubber tubing to the monitored volume, from which it goes to the drain. The flow rate is controlled by adjusting a clamp on the tubing downstream from the monitored volume, and the flow rate is determined by measuring the time necessary to collect a given volume of liquid. Injections are made from a syringe directly into the tubing upstream from the monitored volume. The scanner monitors the volume of interest through a collimator, and a continuous record is made by the recorder.

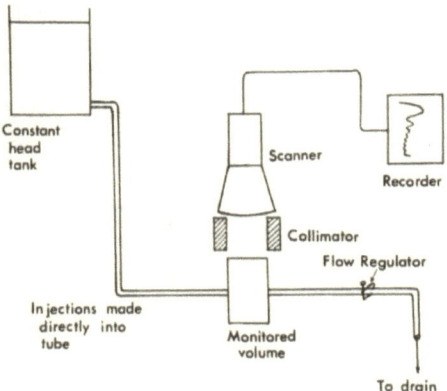

FIG. A-2. Experimental arrangement for model studies to test the basic flow equation.

One of the more interesting results of the analysis leading to the basic flow equation is that this relation should apply for any type of flow pattern existing in the monitored volume. Three different types of experimental models with widely different flow patterns were utilized as monitored volumes in the studies to provide a check of this prediction.

Glass tubes of fairly large size and packed with glass beads were utilized as one type of model. The liquid that flows through such packing follows a tortuous path, and it appears as though the radioactive material is carried through the tube as a front. Thus, this model approximates *rod-like flow*. This model should serve fairly well to describe flow through organs such as the lungs and muscle that contain mainly capillaries.

Glass tubes of lesser diameter which were free of glass beads or other obstructions were used as a model of another type of flow. At low flow rates the flow is *laminar*; the material in the vicinity of the wall is slowed down by the drag of the wall and the fluid near the center of the tube flows at a correspondingly faster rate. Such a model might be expected to approximate flow through large veins and arteries.

A small beaker was equipped with inlet and outlet tubes of small diameter to provide a model of flow through pools of fluid. A magnetic mixer was also provided to give better mixing and thus more closely approximate the mathematical ideal of *perfect mixing*. Such a flow pattern will differ markedly from both models described previously and might be expected to approximate flow conditions as they exist in the two chambers of the heart and in other large pools of blood in the body.

The three models just described (packed tube, empty tube, and stirred beaker) were used in tests of the basic equations as discussed below. In all cases the experiments confirmed that the basic equation is indeed independent of the experimental model used in the investigation.

Recall that the basic flow equation predicts that the area under the time-activity curve, A, is proportional to the net amount of radioactivity injected, I, and the monitored volume, V_M, and is inversely proportional to the volumetric flow rate, F.

$$A = \alpha I \, \frac{V_M}{F} \tag{20}$$

The predicted direct proportionality between area, A, and the injected dose, I, was tested using both a packed tube and a stirred beaker. In each set of experiments the flow rate, F, volume, V_M, and geometrical arrangement between the scanner and the monitored volume, α, were maintained constant. The results conclusively support the basic equation as illustrated in Figure A-3.

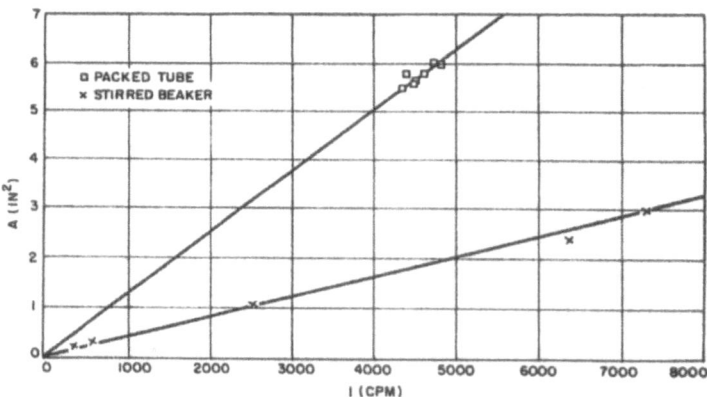

FIG. A-3. Experimental verification of direct proportionality between the area under a time-activity curve (A) and the net injected dosage (I).

In checking the predicted direct proportionality between area A, and monitored volume, V_M, it was necessary to arrange the equipment so that the geometric factor, α, was essentially independent of volume. This was accomplished by using a packed tube and viewing a portion of the tube perpendicular to the axis through a slit formed by lead shielding. Collimation was used to minimize parallax effects on monitored volume definition. Figure A-4 shows a drawing of this particular experimental apparatus.

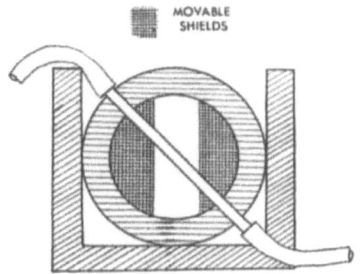

FIG. A-4. Glass tube with movable shielding on scanner collimator designed to permit variation of monitored volume.

The monitored volume was varied by changing the slit width. The result of these experiments substantiates the linear relation between area and monitored volume as illustrated in Figure A-5.

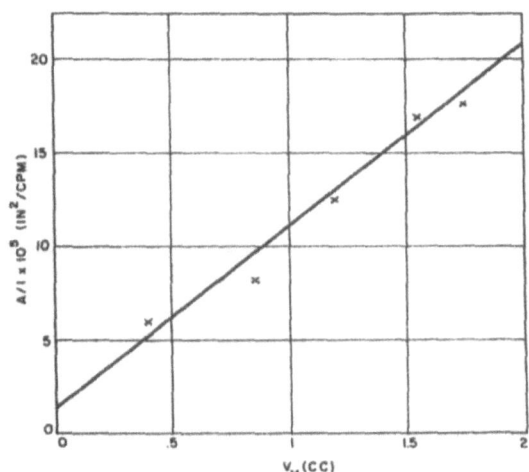

FIG. A-5. Experimental verification of the predicted linear relation between area under time-activity curves (A) and volume (V_M).

Note that the straight line does not pass through the origin because the shielding was not complete, as evidenced by the fact that injections with the slit entirely closed yielded a non-zero scanner reading and therefore a finite area. Note also that the ratio A / I is plotted as the ordinate because it was not practical to insure injection of exactly the same net amount of radioactive material in each experiment. Such plotting is justified by the linear relation between A and I as illustrated in Figure A-3.

According to the basic flow equation, the area is inversely proportional to the flow rate. This relation was checked in packed tubes and mixed beaker models. The results obtained on both models definitely substantiate the basic flow equation, as is illustrated by typical results plotted in Figure A-6.

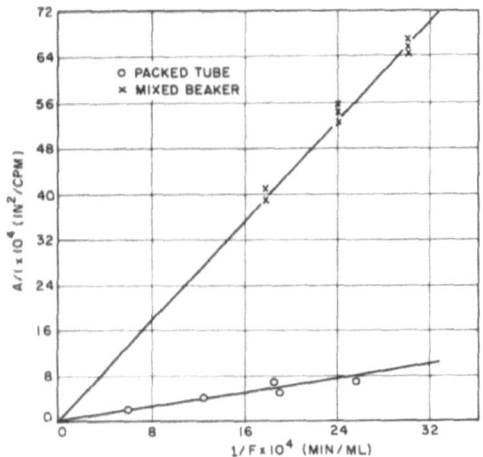

FIG. A-6. Experimental verification of the predicted linear relation between area (A) and the inverse flow rate (I / F).

In addition to checking the predicted dependence of area on injected dose, I, monitored volume, V_M, and flow rate, F, other factors which should not influence the basic relation were also checked. For instance, the distance from the point of injection in the tubing to the monitored volume has a decided influence on the shape of the count rate vs. time curve. As the injection distance is increased, the maximum count rate is diminished and the curve changes, the total area remains constant, independent of injection distance as long as the volume and flow rate are maintained constant. Typical data are presented in Figure A-7.

Other factors that were investigated and found to have no influence on the predicted relation between area, dose, volume, and flow rate include rate of mixing in the mixed beaker, tubing size leading from the injection point to the monitored volume, and initial concentration and volume of the injected bolus. As might be expected, these factors did influence the shape and relative times of the curves.

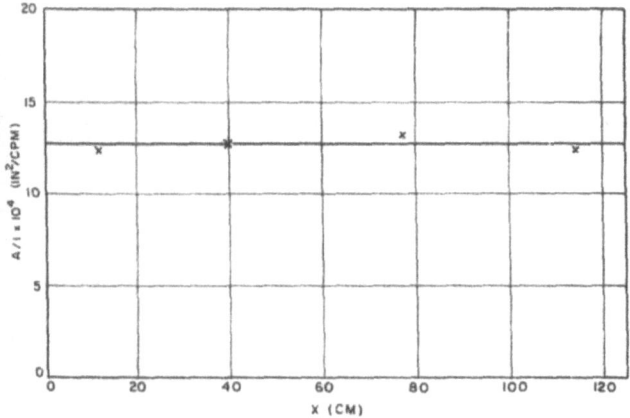

FIG. A-7. Experimental verification of the predicted independence of area (*A*) on injection distance (*X*).

The difficulty of determining the geometric factor, α, prevented a direct check of the basic flow equation and limits its direct application. The most useful techniques involve methods that permit elimination of the geometric factor from the relation which is utilized. Such elimination is relatively easy when one deals with injections into a closed, recycling system. Consider the diagrammatic representation in Figure A-8.

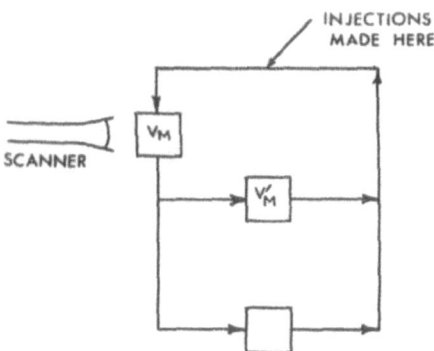

FIG. A-8. Surface monitoring to determine the flow rate in a closed system.

The scanner is placed over the monitored volume, V_M, with fixed geometrical location. A suitable tracer substance is injected into the stream leading to the monitored volume. A continuous record of the scanner reading is made until an equilibrium reading, E, is obtained. Equilibrium is obtained as a result of continual recycling of the radioactive substance, but it is necessary to exclude any effects of recycling in determining the area under the curve. The volumetric flow rate through the monitored organ, F, is calculable from a knowledge of the area under the time-activity curve (excluding recycle), A, the equilibrium reading, E, and the total volume of the closed system, V_t.

$$F = \frac{EV_t}{A} \tag{32}$$

The total volume, V_t, can be determined by use of the dilution technique previously described.

The mathematical justification follows from an application of the basic flow equation in rearranged form:

$$F = \frac{\alpha I V_M}{A} \tag{33}$$

At equilibrium, the scanner sees the same volume, which is filled with fluid of uniform concentration, $C = I/V_t$, where I is the total injected dose and V_t is the total volume:

$$E = \alpha C V_M = \frac{\alpha I}{V_t} V_M \tag{34}$$

Eliminating $\alpha I V_M$ between Equations 33 and 34 yields Equation 32.

Since it is not always practical to inject directly into a stream that flows to the monitored volume without branching, it would be convenient to be able to determine flow rate through volumes that receive only a portion of the injected sample. Sometimes the basic flow equation is used to consider the possibility of determining the flow rate through a volume V'_M in a branch following V_M by placing the monitor over V'_M as in Figure A-8. The basic flow equation applies for the branched flow:

$$F' = \frac{\alpha' I' V'_M}{A'} \tag{35}$$

where primes are used to indicate flow rate and dose passing through the monitored volume V'_M. A' is the area (excluding recycle) obtained from such a determination. The equilibrium reading is related to the total injected dose, I, rather than to the portion that branches into this particular monitored volume.

$$E' = \alpha' \frac{I}{V_t} V'_M \qquad (36)$$

By substituting Equation 36 into Equation 35 $\alpha V'_M$ is eliminated.

$$F' = \frac{E'V_t I'}{A'I} \qquad (37)$$

The development of the basic flow equation was based in a large measure on the assumption that the radioactive substance is uniformly mixed throughout the transporting fluid; it is also reasonable, therefore, to assume that the amount that flows through the branch, I', and the total dose, I, will be in proportion to the branched and unbranched flows, i.e.,

$$\frac{I'}{I} = \frac{F'}{F} \qquad (38)$$

By the substitution of this relation into Equation 37, I' and I are eliminated but the branched flow rate, F', is *also* eliminated. Solving the resulting relation for F yields

$$F = \frac{E'}{A'} V_t \qquad (39)$$

Thus one is forced to the conclusion that the total volume, V_t, together with the equilibrium count rate, E', and the area under the time-activity curve, A', in a volume downstream from a branching determine the flow rate in the *unbranched* portion of the system. However, determinations of flow in branches can be obtained by correct interpretation of simultaneous measurements made in different parts of closed systems and will be discussed later.

Interpretation of simultaneous measurements is in general based on solution of the *differential flow equation*. In the following paragraphs, the differential flow equation is developed, and its application to the interpretation of time-activity curves obtained with a single monitor is discussed.

Consider a monitored volume with inflow and outflow as shown in Figure A-9. If the amount of radioactive decay that occurs inside the monitored volume is negligible, then the principle of conservation of matter can be applied. This basic principle may be expressed as follows:

$$\text{Accumulation} = \text{input} - \text{output} \qquad (40)$$

In this case we are considering the radioactive substance and therefore the rate of accumulation is $dI/d\theta$ where θ stands for time. The rate of input is F_iC_i, and the rate of output is F_oC_o.

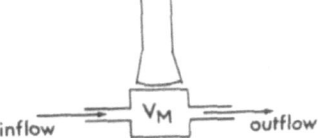

FIG. A-9. General model of a monitored volume with inflow and outflow.

Thus:

$$\frac{dI}{d\theta} = F_iC_i - F_oC_o \tag{41}$$

The scanner reading R is assumed to be in direct proportion to I_M, as discussed previously:

$$R = \alpha \, I_M \tag{2}$$

In dealing with this equation it will be convenient to assume that the geometric factor does not vary with time; that the average concentration in the monitored volume, V_M, is equal to that in the total pool volume, V_v, and, further, that the flow rate in, F_i, is equal to the flow rate out F_o. Under these conditions Equation 41 becomes

$$\frac{dR}{d\theta} = \alpha \, \frac{V_M}{V_P} F(C_i - C_o) \tag{42}$$

This is referred to as the basic differential flow equation and it is restricted only as described above. Thus, simultaneous determinations of R, C_i, and C_o as functions of time should permit evaluation of F (or more correctly, evaluation of the ratio F/V), which possibility is discussed in more detail in a later section. Here we shall consider certain restricted solutions to the basic differential flow equation that aid in the interpretation of time-activity curves obtained with a single monitor.

In a prior paragraph of this chapter a method of determining the volume of an organ by direct injection into that organ was discussed, leading to the result

$$V_M = V_t \frac{E}{R_{max}} \tag{16}$$

66

It was noted that a complete time-activity curve was not required in this determination since only the maximum and equilibrium scanner readings were utilized. However, the complete determination does yield an estimate of the flow rate through the monitored volume. In this connection it is important to understand that the basic flow equation, $A = \alpha I \dfrac{V_M}{F}$, does not apply in cases of direct injection because the radioactive material will not have to travel the entire distance from the inlet to the outlet and therefore will have a residence time distribution differing markedly from that of the transporting fluid. In making use of the complete time-activity curve to estimate the flow rate: (1) The injection is made directly into the monitored volume as previously described and care is taken to insure that the entire pool and nothing else is monitored; (2) The slope, S, is determined from a straight line drawn through the data points plotted as ln R vs. θ (or alternatively from a lot of R vs. θ on semilogarithmic graph paper); (3) The flow rate is calculated as follows:

$$F_M = -\frac{SV_t E}{R_{max}} \qquad (43)$$

where, as before, V_t is the total blood volume, E is the equilibrium count rate, and R_{max} is the maximum recorded count rate.

The mathematical justification of this procedure illustrates application of the basic differential flow equation, Equation 42. In case of direct injection with negligible recycle $C_i = 0$ and the differential flow equation reduces to

$$\frac{dR}{d\theta} = -\alpha \frac{V_m}{V_p} FC_o \qquad (44)$$

In order to solve this relation it is further assumed that the monitored volume is perfectly mixed and therefore of uniform concentration throughout. Under such conditions

$$R = \alpha C_o V_M \qquad (45)$$

and substitution of this relation into Equation 44 yields

$$\frac{dR}{d\theta} = -\frac{F}{V_p} R \qquad (46)$$

This is a first-order, separable, differential equation, the solution of which is:

$$l\,n\,R = -\left(\frac{F}{V_P}\right)\theta + k' \tag{47}$$

where k' is a constant of integration. The equation is thus of the form

$$Y = S\theta + k' \tag{48}$$

and therefore the slope $S = -\left(\dfrac{F}{V_P}\right)$ can be determined as described above.

Substitution of this expression for the slope into equation 16 and rearrangement yield

$$F = -SV_t \frac{V_P}{V_M} \frac{E}{R_{max}} \tag{48a}$$

If the monitor is carefully positioned, the pool volume, V_p, and the monitored volume, V_M, are identical so that Equation 48a reduces to Equation 43. The experimental time-activity curve will contain a maximum because of injection and instrument limitations. Such a maximum is not in keeping with this theoretical equation. Recycle will also affect the results because it eventually establishes the value of E. Therefore, the model is most applicable shortly *after* the maximum is reached and before recycle appears. The experimental data obtained in this particular range, then, should be weighted heavily in determining the slope, S.

The above development predicts an exponential decline in the curve based on direct injection, perfect mixing, and negligible recycle effects. Thus exponential extrapolation can be applied in this case to establish the curve as if there were no recycle. Exponential extrapolation does not apply in all cases.

Consider now the usual case in which injection is made into the stream which flows into the monitored volume. Here the basic flow equation applies and the flow rate can be estimated by application of Equation 32 in case of a closed system. Application of this equation requires estimation of the area under the time-activity curve in the absence of recycle effects and therefore generally requires some type of extrapolation technique. Exponential extrapolation often leads to erroneous results, especially when a major portion of the downslope coincides with recycle effects or is influenced by the monitoring of another volume which happens to be in view of the scanner. A simple solution of the basic differential flow equation provides the basis for an extrapolation technique that appears to offer several advantages.

Consider that a time-activity curve has been obtained, as illustrated in Figure A-10, and it is desirable to estimate the downslope accurately. It is anticipated that other volumes are being monitored during the downstroke and that recycle effects are also important *but* that the upslope and maximum are formed in absence of such effects.

1.   A straight-line extrapolation is made to the baseline from the upslope so as to eliminate the initial part of the curve. In general this straight line will be drawn so as to coincide with the point of inflection of the upslope.

2.   The time at which R_{max} occurs is estimated, and the time interval between the intersection of the straight line with the baseline and the peak time is established (θ').

3.   A value of Z is calculated from a prior knowledge (or estimate) of the ratio F/V_p.

4.   A series of time ratios, θ'/θ' (where θ is measured from the base point established in paragraph 1 above), is obtained from Figure A-11 for various percentages of the peak height, R/R_{max}, using the value of Z calculated by Equation 49. Corresponding values of activity, R, and time, θ, are plotted on the time-activity curve (Figure A-10).

5.   A smooth line is drawn through these points, thereby establishing the downslope using data obtained from the upslope and maximum region only.

6.   Some adjustment of Z may be required, thereby necessitating repetition of the calculation.

$$Z \equiv \frac{\theta'F}{V_p} \tag{49}$$

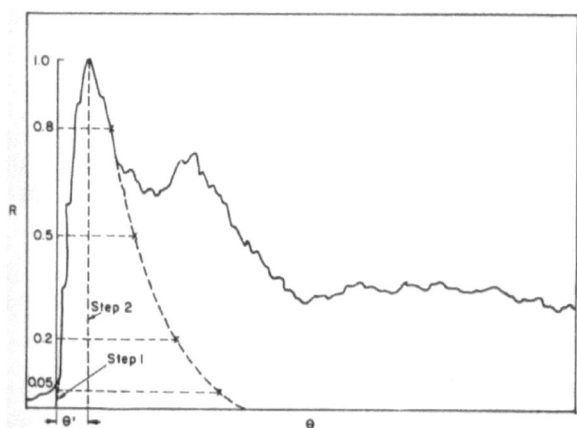

FIG. A-10. Typical time-activity curve illustrating estimation of downslope.

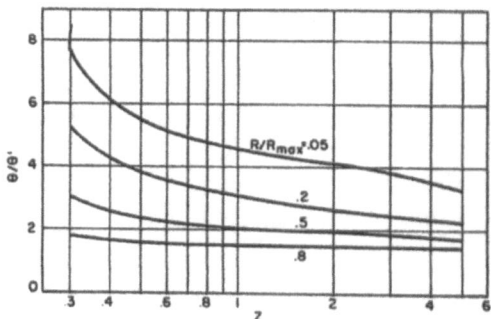

FIG. A-11. Plot used to determine downslope from a knowledge of $Z = \theta'F/V$.

The justification of this procedure is in part theoretical and in part experimental. The theoretical part begins with the basic differential flow equation (Equation 42) and incorporates the assumption of perfect mixing as discussed in connection with the analysis of direct injection. In this case radioactive material flows into the volume and therefore the C_i term remains. The resulting equation is rearranged to yield the following form:

$$\frac{dR}{d\theta} + \frac{F}{V_p} R = \alpha \frac{V_M}{V_p} FC_i \qquad (50)$$

The solution of this first-order, linear, differential equation depends on the precise manner in which the input concentration varies with time; i.e., on $C_i(\theta)$. Such relations can be fairly complicated. In order to avoid undue mathematical complexity the simplest possible input function is chosen as the basis of further development of this model. This function has only two possible values, C_b and zero, as illustrated by the solid line in Figure A-12. The function is expressed mathematically by Equations 51-53.

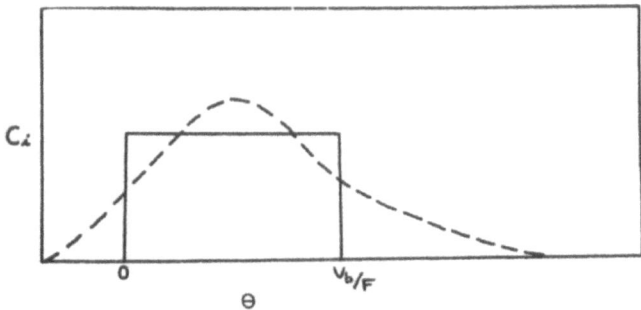

FIG. A-12. Inlet concentration curves for uniform (—) and non-uniform (....) boluses.

For $\theta < 0$;

$$C_i = 0 \qquad (51)$$

For $0 < \theta < \dfrac{V_b}{F}$;

$$C_i = C_b = \dfrac{I}{V_b} \qquad (52)$$

For $\theta > \dfrac{V_b}{F}$;

$$C_i = 0 \qquad (53)$$

where V_b is defined as the volume of the bolus of uniform concentration C_b.

This model, based on the assumptions of perfect mixing and an input consisting of a bolus of uniform concentration C_b and volume V_b, yields the following equations relating R to θ for time intervals corresponding to those of Equations 51-53.

For $\theta < 0$;

$$R = 0 \qquad (54)$$

For $0 < \theta < \dfrac{V_b}{F}$;

$$R = \frac{\alpha I \, V_M}{V_b}\left[1 - \exp\left(-\frac{F\theta}{V_p}\right)\right] \quad (55)$$

For $\theta > \dfrac{V_b}{F}$;

$$R = \frac{\alpha I \, V_M}{V_b}\left[1 - \exp\left(\frac{V_b}{V_p}\right)\right]\exp\left[-\frac{F}{V_p}\left(\theta = \frac{V_b}{F}\right)\right] \quad (56)$$

From these relations it follows that the maximum value of R occurs when $\theta = \dfrac{V_b}{F}$. Therefore, the characteristic bolus volume, V_b, can be estimated by determining the time to the maximum, θ', if the flow rate is known.

$$V_b = F\theta' \quad (57)$$

Note also that Equation 56 has the same general form as Equation 47 in that $\theta > \dfrac{V_b}{F}, C_i = 0,,$ which is the condition that was applied in developing Equation 47. It is interesting to observe, too, that integration of Equations 55 and 56 to evaluate the area under the time-activity curve, A, yields the basic flow relation.

Equations 55 and 56 relate the count rate, R, to many factors. In presenting a plot of these relations it is convenient to assume that $V_p = V_m$ and to present them in dimensionless form using the terms R/R_{max}, θ/θ', and the dimensionless group Z.

$$Z = \frac{\theta' F}{V_p} = \frac{V_b}{V_p} = \frac{V_b}{V_M} \quad (58)$$

Substitution of the correct values into Equations 55 and 56 yields

For $0 < \dfrac{\theta}{\theta'} < 1$;

$$\frac{R}{R_{max}} = \frac{1 - \exp\left(-Z\,\frac{\theta}{\theta'}\right)}{1 - \exp\left(-Z\right)} \qquad (59)$$

For $\dfrac{\theta}{\theta'} > 1$;

$$\frac{R}{R_{max}} = \exp\left[-Z\left(\frac{\theta}{\theta'} - 1\right)\right] \qquad (60)$$

The equations are shown in Figure A-13.

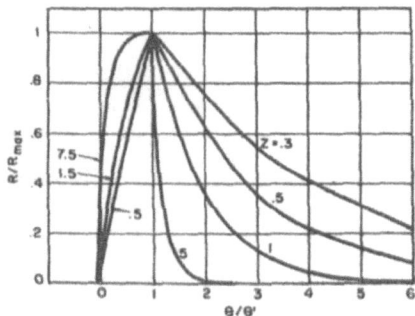

FIG. A-13. Dimensionless plot of Equations 55 and 58 with $Z = \theta' F / V_M$ as a parameter.

The development predicts that the slope will have a maximum value at $\theta = 0$; that a cusp will be formed at the top; and that the downslope will be exponential. None of these predictions are in direct correspondence with experimental observations. Instead, the experimental curves are similar but not identical in form to Equations 59 and 60. The input function C, is shaped more like the dashed line in Figure A-12 than like the rectangle which was assumed in the development of the model. One might choose to assume that all such inputs can be approximated as uniform boluses independent of their actual form. The method of extrapolating the upslope from the point of inflection as previously described, then, serves to bring the experimental data into closer correspondence with the results obtained by detailed consideration of the mathematical model. One would not expect direct correspondence between theory and experiment; therefore, the results of experimental determinations were used in preparing the curves presented in Figure A-11.

73

Briefly, many experimental determinations were made following injection of radioactive tracer material into the stream leading to a monitored volume of a physical model. The upslope was adjusted by drawing a line from the inflection point to the baseline as previously described. The value of θ' thus determined and the value of R_{max} obtained from the curve were used to calculate experimental values of θ/θ' and R/R_{max}. These values for all experimental curves were then plotted on a single sheet of graph paper. Values of Z were calculated from direct measurement of F and V and from values of θ' determined as described above. The solid lines on Figure A-14 result from smoothing the various results. In comparing Figures A-13 and A-14, it is interesting to note their striking similarity, especially with regard to the parametric dependence on the dimensionless term Z. It is also interesting to note that the theoretically predicted and experimentally observed influence of Z on the downslope curves is in agreement, whereas in case of the upslope they are not. This disagreement may result from the method of establishing the initial values of the upslope or may result from the fact that the bolus is not of uniform concentration. The agreement on the downslope side is encouraging and thus Figure A-11 was developed from the smoothed curves of Figure A-14, to serve as a basis for extrapolating downslopes in the manner previously described.

Since *all* experimental curves were included in preparing Figure A-14, use was made of data obtained with models approximating perfect mixing, rod-like flow, and laminar flow. This apparent independence of flow model type is encouraging and contributes to the generality of application of this technique for downslope extrapolation. Thus, an extremely simple mathematical model yielded a basis for correlating experimental data and provides one means of estimating flow through branches which will be discussed in detail in Appendix E, on coronary blood flow.

Mathematical models have also been developed based on rod-like flow and laminar flow through the monitored volume. These developments suggest methods of estimating flow rates through monitored volumes but would be useful only if very smooth curves were obtained. In application to clinical studies, neither the experimental data nor the models justify such refinements. However, the rod-like flow model does play an important role in the interpretation of simultaneous determinations and will therefore be considered in more detail in a later section of this chapter.

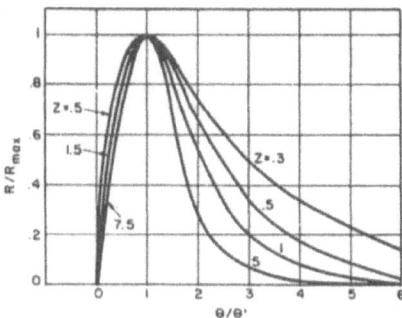

FIG. A-14. Smoothed curves produced by scaling experimental time-activity curves obtained on various physical models.

CLEARANCE DETERMINATIONS. Previous sections of this chapter have dealt with the interpretation of time-activity curves obtained when injection is made either directly into the monitored volume or directly into a stream that flows into the monitored volume. Interpretation of such curves is based on the assumption that transfer of the radioactive material from the vascular to the extravascular system is not significant. In studies of clearance rate a major part of the radioactive material is injected into the extravascular system and is only transported from the monitored volume following transfer to the vascular system. Thus, power interpretation of data obtained in clearance studies requires that the rate of transfer between the two systems be considered.

Choice of a suitable radioactive substance is of primary importance. In brief, the distribution coefficient of the substance between the vascular and extravascular systems should greatly favor the vascular system and the transfer of the material between the two systems should be as rapid as possible. The material is injected into the extravascular portion of the monitored volume and a continuous record is made of count rates. As was the case with interpretation of the results obtained upon direct injection into the fluid portion of a monitored volume, discussed previously, the negative slope, S, of a plot of $ln\ R$ vs. θ (or of R vs. θ on semilogarithmic paper) is a direct measure of the *rate of clearance* as determined by the combined influence of flow rate through the capillaries *and* rate of transfer from the extravascular to the vascular system. Only if the rate of transfer between systems is extremely rapid will the clearance factor, S, be related to the flow rate, F, in a simple manner. The mathematical development which follows as justification of this method of determining a clearance factor will hopefully clarify this point.

75

The model that serves as the basis for the mathematical analysis is illustrated in Figure A-15.

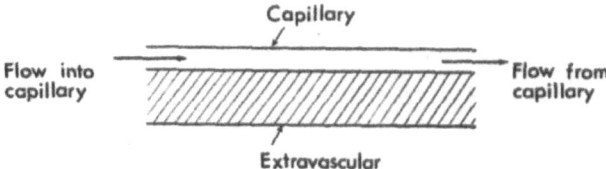

FIG. A-15. Model for mathematical analysis of clearance studies.

In the model the monitored volume includes both the capillary and extravascular parts, and for this total system the basic differential flow equation describing the dependence of the rate of change of count rate on the inlet and outlet flows (Equation 42) applies. Since in most clearance studies the volume of blood that is monitored is very small, the equilibrium count rate and recycle effects are negligible. Under these conditions little or no radioactive material enters the system after the initial injection and therefore $C_i = 0$. Therefore, Equation 42 reduces to

$$\frac{dR}{d\theta} = -\alpha F C_o \qquad (61)$$

This equation is identical to the one developed in the initial part of the analysis of direct injection into the monitored fluid, but the circumstances are quite different. Whereas the assumption of perfect mixing was applied in that particular case to provide a rapid and useful solution, such an assumption is unrealistic in application to the present case because the monitored volume consists of two distinct regions. The transfer between the two regions must be taken into account in relating C_o to R in order to obtain a solution to Equation 61.

The transfer from the extravascular to the vascular system is considered to occur across an interface between the two phases. The rate of transfer is assumed to be proportional to the area available for such transfer and to the difference in concentration of the radioactive material in the two phases in relation to the equilibrium distribution. Expressed in mathematical terms:

$$\dot{I} = kA(\beta C' - C) \qquad (62)$$

where $\dot{I}$ is the rate of transfer of radioactive material from the extravascular to the vascular system, A is the area available for transfer between the two phases, β is the distribution coefficient, and C' is the concentration in the extravascular system in the region of transfer. C refers to the concentration in the vascular system in the region of transfer, and k is a proportionality factor which is sometimes referred to as a mass-transfer coefficient. The distribution coefficient β is the ratio of concentrations in the two phases *under conditions of equilibrium*, (C/C'), and, as a result, the rate of transfer is zero at equilibrium.

It is assumed that the concentration of material flowing into the system is zero, and it is desired to relate the outlet concentration, C_o, to R in order to solve Equation 61. Thus, the important variation of C from inlet to outlet is taken into account by reference to a different element of the vascular system. Considerable simplification results in this development if it is assumed that the radioactive material in the vascular portion of the total monitored volume is small and does not contribute materially to the scanner reading, R. Under these conditions the variation of C with time is ignored in order to obtain an ordinary differential equation relating C to position within the capillary, x.

$$\frac{dC}{dx} = -\frac{kA_t}{FL}(\beta C' - C) \tag{63}$$

where A_t is the total area for transfer between phases contained in the entire monitored volume and L is the length of the capillary over which the integration is to be performed.

A further simplification is made by assuming that the concentration of radioactive material in the extravascular system is uniform throughout, i.e., $C' \neq f(x)$. This assumption, plus consideration of k and β as constants, permits separation and integration of Equation 63 yielding a relation between C_o and C':

$$C_o = \beta C' \left[1 - \exp\left(\frac{kA_t}{F}\right)\right] \tag{64}$$

For a uniform concentration C' in the extravascular volume, V'

$$R = \alpha C' V' \tag{65}$$

The monitored volume, V_M, is related to the volume of the extravascular system, V', by assuming the blood volume to be negligible.

$$V' = V_M \tag{65a}$$

Combination of Equations 64, 65, and 65a to eliminate C' and substitution into Equation 61 yields

$$\frac{dR}{d\theta} = -\beta \frac{F}{V_M} \left[1 - \exp\left(\frac{-kA_t}{F}\right) \right] R \qquad (66)$$

Separation and integration yields

$$ln\, R = -\beta \frac{F}{V_M} \left[1 - \exp\left(\frac{-kA_t}{F}\right) \right] \theta + K \qquad (67)$$

where K is a constant of integration. Thus, the slope, S, or clearance rate, as determined from a plot of $ln\, R$ vs. θ is as follows:

$$S = -\beta \frac{F}{V_M} \left[1 - \exp\left(\frac{-kaV_M}{F}\right) \right] \qquad (68)$$

where α is the surface area for transfer per unit volume. Note that the ratio of flow rate to volume, F/V_M, enters this relation both as a multiplying factor and as a divisor within the exponential term. In addition, the clearance rate, S, is dependent, in part, on the transfer rate terms k and a. As a result, the clearance rate will be directly proportional to F/V_M *only* if the ratio kaV_M/F is very large, i.e., at relatively high transfer rates. At low values of this ratio the clearance rate S becomes *independent of flow rate* as the flow rate increases. As a result, interpretation of changes in clearance factors in terms of flow rates can lead to erroneous conclusions.

USE OF SIMULTANEOUS DETERMINATIONS

The preceding parts of this chapter deal with the interpretation of equilibrium activity measurements and time-activity curves obtained with a single monitor-recorder to yield information with regard to volume of and flow rate through various organs. If injections can be made directly into the monitored volume or into a stream so that the entire injection passes through the monitored volume, it is comparatively easy to determine both volume and flow rates using a single surface monitor. However, it is often much more convenient to inject the radioactive material so that a branch occurs and only a portion of the tracer passes through the organ. In these cases it is necessary to make simultaneous determinations; either time-activity determinations over two or more organs or a combination of time-activity curves together with time concentration determinations. The rest of this chapter is devoted to analyzing data of this nature.

DETERMINATION OF RELATIVE VOLUMES. Consider that flow occurs through two volumes in sequence, as illustrated in Figure A-16. If a suitable tracer material is injected into the stream entering volume V_1 and time-activity curves are obtained for the individual volumes in such a way that the geometric and scanner factors, α_1 and α_2, are identical, then the volumes V_1 and V_2 are in direct proportion to the areas under their respective curves.

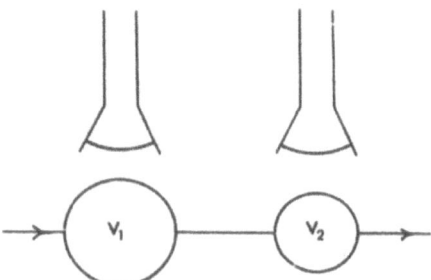

FIG. A-16. Flow through two volumes in sequence.

$$\frac{V_1}{V_2} = \frac{A_1}{A_2} \tag{69}$$

The mathematical justification of this relation follows by application of the basic flow equation:

$$A_1 = \frac{\alpha_1 I_1 V_1}{F_1} \tag{70}$$

$$A_2 = \frac{\alpha_2 I_2 V_2}{F_2} \tag{71}$$

The total doses, I_1 and I_2, and the total flow rates, F_1 and F_2, are identical because the flow occurs in sequence. Therefore, these terms cancel when the ratio A_1/A_2 is obtained from Equations 70 and 71.

$$\frac{A_1}{A_2} = \frac{\alpha_1 V_1}{\alpha_2 V_2} \tag{72}$$

If the geometric and scanner factors can be made identical, Equation 72 reduces to Equation 69. In general it will be very difficult to insure the identity to these factors.

Equations 69 and 72 apply equally well to simultaneous determinations in which only a portion of the injection passes through the second volume because of a branch. This arrangement is illustrated in Figure A-17.

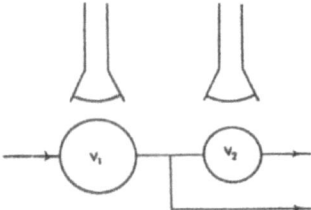

FIG. A-17. Flow through two volumes with branching between.

Equations 70 and 71 apply in this case but $I_1 \neq I_2$ and $F_1 \neq F_2$. However, the principle of uniform branching (discussed in connection with Equation 38) applies, and therefore

$$\frac{I_1}{F_1} \frac{I_2}{F_2} \tag{73}$$

Thus, these ratios cancel in the development of Equation 72 from Equations 70 and 71 in the case of branched flow.

FLOW RATE DETERMINATIONS IN BRANCHED FLOW. As developed in a preceding section the differential flow equation relates the monitored reading, R, to the flow rate, F, and the inlet and outlet concentrations, C_i and C_o.

$$\frac{dR}{d\theta} = \alpha F (C_i - C_o) \tag{42}$$

Thus, in theory at least, simultaneous determinations of R, C_i and C_o as functions of time would permit determination of F through any organ. This general approach will be discussed briefly in a later paragraph but the majority of the section will be devoted to the use of models to facilitate interpretation of simultaneous determinations.

First consider that a time-activity curve is determined by surface monitoring over an organ in which rod-like flow is approximated and further that the inlet concentration, C_i, is simultaneously determined. These two determinations are represented by solid lines in Figure A-18.

The ratio of the organ volume to flow rate, V_p/F, can be estimated in the following manner as illustrated in Figure A-18:

1. The time at which the maximum occurs on the $R(\theta)$ curve is determined, and a vertical line is drawn at that point.

2. At the point of intersection of this vertical line and the $C_i(\theta)$ curve, a horizontal line is drawn.

3. The actual time between the intersections of this horizontal line and the $C_i(\theta)$ curve is the average residence time λ_{ave}.

The value of λ_{ave} is numerically equal to the ratio $\dfrac{V_p}{F}$.

$$\lambda_{ave} = \frac{V_p}{F} \qquad (74)$$

Thus, a prior knowledge of V_p permits estimation of F, and likewise a prior knowledge of F permits estimation of V_p. This interpretation is subject to the restriction of rod-like flow through the volume and thus might serve as the basis for interpretation of time-activity curves obtained on the lungs, coronary artery, and other such organs where the flow is predominantly through capillaries. It would not be expected to apply when flow occurs through large blood pools such as the two heart chambers. This method finds application in estimation of coronary blood flow and will be discussed in detail in Appendix E.

The mathematical justification of this simple procedure is based on two basic principles. First it is noted that at the maximum point on the $R(\theta)$ curve, $dR/d\theta = 0$. As a result, from Equation 42 at the time the maximum occurs,

$$C_i = C_o \qquad (75)$$

This result is independent of any assumptions regarding the nature of flow inside the organ for it is obtained directly from Equation 42 without any additional assumptions.

The second necessary condition for application of the method is based on the concept of rod-like flow. In rod-like flow all particles have exactly the same residence time λ_{ave}, and thus the concentration at the outlet, C_o, is identical to that of the inlet except for the fact that it occurs later in time by the amount λ_{ave}.

$$C_o(\theta) = C_i(\theta - \lambda_{ave}) \qquad (76)$$

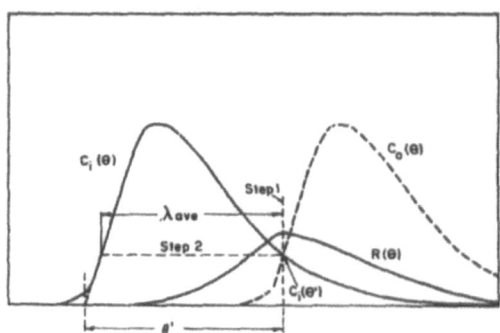

FIG. A-18. Interpretation of simultaneous determinations of volume content [R(θ)] and inlet concentration [C$_i$(θ)].

When one draws a vertical line from R_{max}, a value of C_i is established because the $R(\theta)$ and $C_i(\theta)$ determinations were made simultaneously and therefore have the same time scale. This also establishes a value of $C_o = C_i$ from Equation 75. The output curve is assumed to be identical to that of the input except for a delay time of λ_{ave} and, therefore, the value of λ_{ave} is established by drawing a horizontal line which intersects the upslope of the input curve, $C_i(\theta)$, as illustrated in Figure A-18. A knowledge of one point on the C_o curve together with the complete C_i curve therefore permits establishment of the entire C_o curve, as is also illustrated by the dashed line in Figure A-18. However, it is not generally necessary to establish $C_o(\theta)$ because one is primarily interested in estimating a value of λ_{ave}, which is equal to V_p/F as given by Equation 74.

The application of this procedure to estimate the flow rate through blood pools would not be expected to yield good results because the development is based on the assumption of rod-like flow. For flow through blood pools one might hope to make use of the assumption of perfect mixing in order to determine the ratio V_p/F from simultaneous $R(\theta)$ and $C_i(\theta)$ determinations. Such an analysis is much more complicated in considering a general case and can probably be done only on a repetitive basis with the aid of computers. However, the method is outlined briefly below and followed by a mathematical justification.

1. The time from the start of the $C_i(\theta)$ curve and the $R(\theta)$ curve (which correspond) to the maximum of the $R(\theta)$ curve, θ', is determined. (See Figure A-18.)

2. A value of $C_i(\theta')$—the value of the inlet concentration at the time the maximum in the $R(\theta)$ curve occurs—is also determined.

82

3. A value of F/V_p is found that satisfies the following integral expression:

$$C_i(\theta')=\frac{F}{V_p}\exp\left[-\frac{F\theta'}{V_p}\right]\int_o^{\theta'}C_i(\theta)\exp\left[\frac{F\theta}{V_p}\right]d\theta \qquad (77)$$

Thus a value of θ' as determined from the $R(\theta)$ curve is used in conjunction with the $C_i(\theta)$ curve to establish F/V_p. Some iterative procedure will have to be followed to obtain a value of F/V_p that satisfies the equation, and each iteration will require evaluation of the integral from $\theta = 0$ to the peak time, θ'. If the function $C_i(\theta)$ can be represented in suitable form, an iterative determination can be made rapidly and easily on a repetitive basis by using an electronic computer.

The mathematical justification follows from the basic differential flow equation (Equation 42), in which the assumptions are made that perfect mixing exists in the volume and that $V_M = V_p$.

$$\frac{dR}{d\theta}+\frac{F}{V_p}R=\alpha FC_i \qquad (50)$$

This first-order linear differential equation has the following general solution in terms of the function $C_i(\theta)$

$$R=R(0)\exp\left[-\frac{F\theta}{V_p}\right]+\alpha F\exp\left[-\frac{F\theta}{V_p}\right]\int_o^{\theta}C_i(\theta)\exp\left[\frac{F\theta}{V_p}\right]d\theta \quad(78)$$

by application of standard techniques of solution of such equations. In this equation $R(0)$ is the scanner reading at $\theta = 0$ and this is zero when θ is defined as beginning when the $R(\theta)$ curve first begins.

At the maximum point of the $R(\theta)$ curve, $R = R_{max}$, and for a perfectly mixed volume this is related to C_o by the simple relation

$$R_{max} = \alpha C_o V_p \qquad (79)$$

Equation 75 also applies at the maximum for a perfectly mixed model so that

$$R_{max} = \alpha C_i(\theta') V_p \qquad (80)$$

Application of this relation to eliminate the geometric factor from Equation 78 and substitution of R_{max} for R, zero for $R(0)$, and θ' for θ yields

$$R_{max} = \frac{R_{max}}{C_i(\theta')} \frac{F}{V_p} \exp\left[-\frac{F\theta'}{V_p}\right] \int_0^{\theta'} \exp\left[\frac{F\theta}{V_p}\right] C_i(\theta)d\theta \quad (81)$$

Cancellation of R_{max} and solution for $C_i(\theta')$ yields Equation 77.

If one were to determine $R(\theta)$, $C_i(\theta)$, and $C_o(\theta)$ simultaneously, the basic differential flow equation, Equation 42, could be applied to determine the ratio F/V without any assumptions with regard to the flow characteristics inside the monitored volume as were necessary in treating the rod-like flow and perfectly mixed models in the preceding paragraphs. The equation can be used either in differential or in integral form.

If very accurate determinations of $R(\theta)$ are made and the nature of the experimental curves permits estimates of the slope at a point $dR/d\theta$, the ratio of flow to volume, F/V, is determined as follows:

$$\frac{F}{V_p} = \frac{\left(\dfrac{dR}{d\theta}\right)}{(C_i - C_o)} \frac{\int_0^\infty C_i(\theta)d\theta}{A} \quad (82)$$

where A is the total area under the time-activity curves as previously defined and similarly the integral relation in Equation 82 is the total area under the *entire* time concentration curve. Values of $dR/d\theta$, C_i and C_o must all be determined at the same time.

The mathematical justification of this relation starts with the basic differential flow equation in rearranged form:

$$F = \frac{1}{\alpha} \frac{\dfrac{(dR)}{d\theta}}{(C_i - C_o)} \quad (83)$$

The geometric factor, α, is eliminated from consideration by utilizing two different methods of calculating the total amount of radioactive material that passes through the monitored volume. One method of calculation results from rearrangement of the basic flow equation, Equation 20.

$$I = \frac{AF}{\alpha V_p} \tag{84}$$

One can also relate I to the flow rate and to the inlet concentration function $C_i(\theta)$ as follows:

$$I = F \int_0^\infty C_i(\theta)\,d\theta \tag{85}$$

Solving for α from Equations 84 and 85 yields

$$\alpha = \frac{A}{Vp \int_0^\infty C_i(\theta)\,d\theta} \tag{86}$$

which when substituted into Equation 83 yields Equation 82.

In general, it will be difficult to obtain accurate values of the slope, $Dr/d\theta$, from clinical curves, in which case an integral expression might offer some advantages in terms of accuracy. In the same manner F/V_p can be determined as follows:

$$\frac{F}{V_p} = \frac{R_{max} \int_0^\infty Ci(\theta)\,d\theta}{A\left[\int_0^{\theta'} C_i(\theta)\,d\theta - \int_0^{\theta'} C_o(\theta)\,d\theta\right]} \tag{87}$$

This relation results from direct integration of the differential flow equation (Equation 42) between the limits of $\theta = 0$ and θ' corresponding to the maximum on the time-activity curve.

$$R_{max} - R(0) = \alpha F\left[\int_0^{\theta'} C_i(\theta)\,d\theta - Co(\theta)\,d\theta\right] \tag{88}$$

As discussed previously, $R(0) = 0$ in keeping with the definition of θ'. Substitution of Equation 86 to eliminate α and rearrangement yields Equation 87.

Gunnar Sevelius, MD

APPENDIX B
BLOOD VOLUME

Samuel B. Nadler & John U. Hidalgo

THE CIRCULATING VOLUME OF BLOOD is a mixture of formed elements (red and white cells) and solutes (proteins, crystalloids) in solution (the plasma). This volume is contained within the vascular space, which not only varies in capacity from time to time in a given individual but under certain conditions may allow any and all of the components to escape into the perivascular spaces. The blood volume is the sum of the volume of the plasma and the volume of the cells in the vascular space. A true measure of circulating blood volume requires that both these volumes be measured. For clinical purposes, this is a tedious and often impractical procedure. It is common practice to measure either the red cell volume or the plasma volume and estimate the total blood volume from this value. Such a procedure entails accuracy of technique and an understanding of the limitations of the methods used.

The blood contained in the vascular bed is in *dynamic equilibrium* with its immediate neighbor, the extracellular fluid, and exchanges of substances leaving the blood and returning to it go on constantly. The extracellular fluid is in turn in equilibrium with the intracellular fluid compartment. Figure B-1 indicates that total body water comprises approximately 70 percent of the total body weight and it is so distributed that 5 percent is in the vascular bed, 15 percent in the extracellular fluid compartment, and 50 percent in the body cells. Regulation of the blood volume is largely determined by the balance between fluid in the blood vessels and in the extravascular compartments. (Thus blood volume cannot be considered apart from the body fluid compartments.) When circulating fluid is lost, the extravascular fluid stores are called upon to replenish it (e.g., in dehydration); when the blood volume tends to increase, fluid is transferred to the perivascular spaces or excreted in the urine. The volume of circulating blood is maintained at a surprisingly constant level in health.

The volume of water in the vascular bed and extracellular compartment can be measured by the injection of substances which either do not penetrate cells or do so only to a minor degree; e.g., mannitol, inulin, thiocyanate, and radioactive sodium. When thiocyanate is used to measure this volume it distributes itself evenly throughout the entire volume. A subsequent measure of its concentration in the plasma

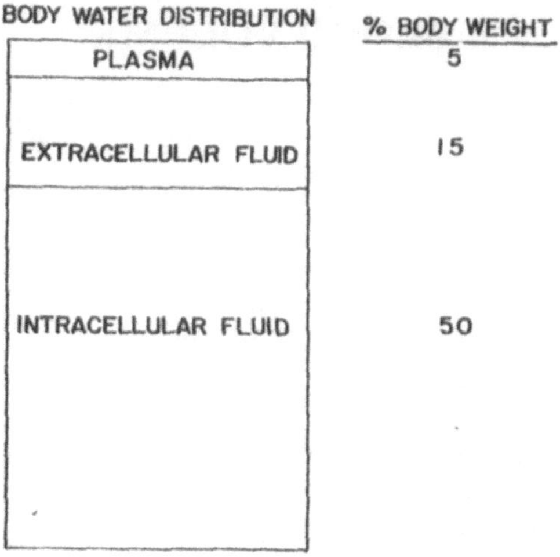

BODY WATER DISTRIBUTION	% BODY WEIGHT
PLASMA	5
EXTRACELLULAR FLUID	15
INTRACELLULAR FLUID	50

FIG. B-1. Body water distribution.

indicates the degree of dilution or the volume of the so-called "thiocyanate space." Antipyrine and water labeled with deuterium or tritium distribute themselves evenly throughout the total body water and may serve to measure this volume.

According to Starling's theory, two main factors governing the movement of fluid out of the vascular bed into the extracellular space and into the capillary bed from this space are osmotic pressure and hydrostatic pressure. In health, the capillary walls behave as membranes of selective permeability, allowing the passage of water and some substances in solution but acting as a barrier to molecules of certain other substances. The membranes of cell walls, capillaries, renal epithelium, and serous cavities are interposed between different concentrations of osmotically active substances.

The capillary membrane is freely permeable to water and molecules of small size, e.g., inorganic salts, urea, glucose. The plasma colloids, albumins, globulins, and fibrinogen are largely barred from leaving the capillary lumen. Studies with I^{131} labeled albumin indicate that some albumin molecules, smallest of the plasma colloids, do leave the vascular bed. The protein is picked up by the lymphatic system and returned to the circulating blood via the thoracic duct.

Because the plasma colloids are contained within the vascular bed on one side of the capillary membrane, they can exert water-pulling power and draw fluid into the vascular bed from the perivascular spaces. This force is referred to as the oncotic pressure of the plasma proteins. In a measure, this force is assisted by the hydrostatic pressure of tissues on the perivascular spaces (tissue pressure), which enhances the movement of fluid and solutes into the capillary bed. The hydrostatic force of arterial blood pressure tends to push fluid out of the vascular bed into the perivascular spaces.

At the arterial end of the capillary, the hydrostatic pressure exerted by blood pressure is about 30 mm Hg, although this varies in different parts of the capillary bed. The hydrostatic pressure of the extracellular fluid (tissue pressure) is approximately 10 mm Hg. Thus the effective hydrostatic pressure at the arterial end of the capillary is 20 mm Hg. This hydrostatic pressure diminishes progressively until at the venous end of the capillary it is about 10 mm, equaling the hydrostatic pressure of the perivascular fluid and resulting in zero effective hydrostatic pressure. High hydrostatic pressure at the arterial end of the capillary tends to increase filtration into the perivascular spaces, whereas the hydrostatic pressure at the venous end of the capillary exerts no such effect.

At the arterial end of the capillary the osmotic pressure of the plasma proteins (oncotic pressure) approximates 25 mm Hg. This force tends to pull water into the capillary bed at the arterial end, and it is opposed by the osmotic pressure of the extracellular fluid, which contains far less protein and approximates 15 mm Hg. Thus, the effective osmotic pressure at the arterial end of the capillary tending to draw fluid into the capillary from the perivascular spaces is 10 mm Hg. The 10 mm Hg effective osmotic pressure is opposed by the effective hydrostatic pressure at the arterial end of the capillary of 20 mm Hg (Figure B-2). The resultant effective pressure favors filtration out of the capillary bed into the perivascular spaces at the arterial end of the capillary. The situation is reversed at the venous end of the capillary. As blood progresses along the capillary bed toward the venous end, loss of filtration fluid progressively raises the concentration of plasma proteins, increasing their water-pulling power. Unopposed by effective hydrostatic pressure, this oncotic pressure favors absorption of fluid from the perivascular spaces into the capillary bed at the venous end of the capillary. The rate of diffusion in both directions across the capillary membrane is enormously high, approximating 1500 liters per minute in a 70 kg man.

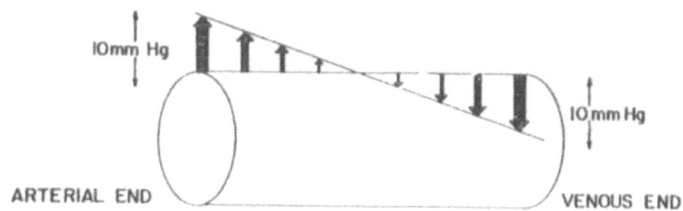

FIG. B-2. Resultant effective capillary pressures.

Changes in blood volume are associated with changes in either hydrostatic pressure or osmotic pressure or both. After hemorrhage, vasoconstriction decreases hydrostatic pressure in the capillary bed, reducing filtration. The osmotic pressure is unchanged, and fluid moves into the vascular bed. Loss of water from the blood in states of dehydration causes the concentration of the plasma proteins to rise. The increased osmotic pressure draws water into the capillary bed from the perivascular spaces. Infusions of large quantities of isotonic salt solution dilute the plasma proteins, decrease the osmotic pressure, and at the same time increase the hydrostatic pressure. Conditions then favor removal of excess fluid from the circulating blood into the perivascular spaces, from which it may later be excreted. Thus the factors of osmosis and hydrostatic pressure play important roles in the regulation of circulating blood volume.

Variations in blood volume under physiologic conditions are known to occur. Long periods of bed rest, standing quietly, exposure to cold, and short bouts of vigorous exercise are associated with decrease in plasma volume chiefly and a net decrease in blood volume. On the other hand, the blood volume is increased with prolonged exercise such as in the training of athletes, exposure to high altitudes, temporary recumbent position, and pregnancy.

In pathologic states, reduction of blood volume is associated with (1) loss of whole blood, hemorrhage, (2) loss of plasma, burns, (3) loss of water, dehydration, (4) marked decrease in red blood cells, severe anemias, and (5) myxedema, mainly due to reduction of red blood cells. Increase in circulating blood volume may be found in (1) hyperthyroidism, (2) congestive heart failure, (3) polycythemia vera, increase mainly of red cells but also of plasma, and (4) leukemia, increase of white cells and plasma.

The effects of hemorrhage on circulating blood volume depend on whether the hemorrhage is from an artery or a vein, on the volume of the hemorrhage, and on the speed with which it is occurring.

After the withdrawal of 500 ml of blood from a blood donor, the blood volume may be restored to normal by the movement of fluid into the vascular bed from the perivascular spaces within an hour. With moderate slow loss of blood—15 percent of the total blood volume—there may be little or no drop in blood pressure, especially if the bleeding is venous. If more than one-third of the blood volume is rapidly lost, the body is usually unable to repair the loss unaided and death may result unless transfusion is given.

Compensation for blood loss is attained by reduction in the capacity of the vascular bed, increase in peripheral resistance and the drawing of fluid from the perivascular spaces into the capillary bed. With large hemorrhage, the marked drop in hydrostatic pressure within the capillaries allows fluid to move into the vessels and dilute the blood. The concentration of red blood cells is reduced, and the plasma proteins in turn are decreased in concentration. Mobilization of protein from protein stores can result in rapid restoration of the serum protein level. The replacement of red blood cells may go on for a period of days or weeks.

Reduction in the size of the vascular bed with maintenance of blood pressure is effected by reflex narrowing (vasoconstriction) of small blood vessels in nonessential areas—the skin, mucous membrane, intestine. This constriction may be enough to maintain adequate venous return and cardiac output. With larger hemorrhage, however, venous return and cardiac output may fall, in which case peripheral resistance occasioned by arteriolar constriction is brought into play. If in spite of these mechanisms the hemorrhage is sufficient to cause fall in arterial blood pressure, entrance of fluid from the perivascular spaces into the blood vessels may help to restore the volume of fluid in the vascular bed. In the effort of the organism to preserve vital centers, the vasoconstrictor effects are noted in pallor of the skin and mucous membranes and coldness of the body surface. In the ultimate vasoconstrictor effort, small arteries, arterioles, metarterioles, precapillary sphincters, and venules are involved. If there is very severe, rapid, massive hemorrhage, capillary reactivity may give place to one of reduced response with the onset of hemorrhagic shock. The smaller vessels dilate while larger vessels remain constricted.

Clinical states with water loss from the organism can be associated with marked change in circulating blood volume. Such dehydration may occur as a result of water deprivation, excessive loss of fluid and electrolyte associated with gastrointestinal disturbances, and salt depletion syndromes associated with gastrointestinal losses of fluids and electrolytes. In severe states of dehydration, inspissation of blood may occur to such an extent that the quantity of circulating blood is inadequate to meet the demands of the organism and exhaustion and collapse can follow.

The history of blood volume measurement is the story of the development of methods of measuring blood volume (110).

Direct methods of measuring blood volume are of purely historical interest. The basic technique was to determine the total amount of hemoglobin after complete bleed-out and washing of the vascular tree with water or plasma. The hemoglobin content of this fluid was then compared to a standard dilution of previously drawn venous blood hemoglobin. Such studies are terminal and of little practical value, but the early work of Welcker in 1854 produced data of surprising accuracy (344). As carried out by Whipple and his co-workers (9), the method was used to check the accuracy of labeling techniques. Indirect methods involve the dilution of labeled red blood cells or labeled plasma substance in the red cell or plasma volume. These methods are available for the determination of blood volume during life. Simultaneous measurement of red cell volume and plasma volume has also been done.

The dilution of labeled red cells as a measure of red cell volume employs a basic procedure of labeling the red blood cells with a tagging material and determining the dilution of the injected tagged cells in the circulating red cell volume of the subject. A variety of substances (including carbon monoxide, Fe^{59}, Cr^{51}, P^{32}, K^{42}) have been used for this purpose. The most common method for measuring red cell volume is the original or modified method of Sterling and Gray (296). The various test substances employed to measure plasma volume had to be selected for their ability to remain in the circulation long enough to allow the recording of adequate measurement data. Dyes were first employed by Keith, Rowntree, and Geraghty (143) in 1915, with the introduction of vital red and brilliant vital red to stain the plasma. With a simple colorimetric method they were able to make numerous basic observations. Other substances used are dextran and albumin tagged with I^{131}.

The best and most commonly used plasma dye today is T-1824 (Evans blue), which was extensively studied by Gregersen and his co-workers. The requirements to be fulfilled by an ideal dye substance are several: the dye must be harmless, diffuse slowly from the bloodstream, color only the plasma, maintain its color in the plasma, not cause hemolysis, and be capable of mixing uniformly with the plasma. Since it leaves the circulation rather slowly in normal persons (3 percent in ten minutes), a reasonably accurate estimate of dilution in plasma can be obtained from a sample taken ten minutes after dye injection (109). For greater accuracy serial determinations of dye concentration and extrapolating the disappearance curve to zero are essential. T-1824 estimations are interfered with by lipemia or hemolysis. Additional disadvantages are discoloration of the skin and conjunctivae and the inability to do repeated determinations at short intervals of time because of the difficulties in estimating residual dye. I^{131} tagged albumin is not affected by hemolysis or lipemia and does not cause staining of tissues. Repeat determinations can be done at short intervals with easily determined residual radioactivity in the control blood.

The simultaneous measurement of red cell volume and plasma volume gives a true figure for circulating blood volume. The usual method of carrying out the technique is to use a red cell tag (P^{32}, Cr^{51}) and a plasma tag (T-1824 or I^{131}). Gray and Frank (105) used an ingenious technique employing Cr^{51}-$Cr^{51}Cl_3$ for the simultaneous red cell and plasma tagging. Such measurements give an estimate of the body hematocrit, and the ratio of the corrected venous hematocrit to the body hematocrit is easily estimated. Accuracy can be achieved with meticulous attention to technical details.

Isotopic methods have much to recommend them. Isotopes are inexpensive, readily available, harmless when properly used, easily identified in body fluids, and they can be readily measured. The superiority of isotope methods over dye methods is evidenced by greater accuracy (366) and the opportunity to do repeated determinations at short intervals. When I^{131} human serum albumin is injected, the injected albumin will mix completely with blood within two minutes (362, 187). The extent of dilution of tagged albumin in the circulating plasma is a true measure of the volume of the plasma, provided (1) dilution and mixing are uniform and (2) there is no loss of iodinated albumin into the perivascular spaces. It is generally agreed that a ten-minute post-injection sample allows enough time for adequate mixing in most, if not all, clinical states. By this time some of the tagged albumin has left the vascular space to enter the perivascular space. Graphic analysis of the time concentration curve on semilog paper with extrapolation to zero time permits estimation of this loss. Such refinement of calculation is unnecessary for clinical purposes since the loss of I^{131} albumin ten minutes after injection is only 2 to 3 percent (270). In our laboratory, I^{131} human serum albumin is used as the plasma tag, and sodium chromate ($Na_2Cr^{51}O_4$) is used as the red cell tag. Details of the use of these two methods are given below.

TECHNIQUE OF I^{131} HSA BLOOD VOLUME ESTIMATION

Radioactive iodinated human serum albumin as procured from commercial suppliers varies in radioactivity from 200 μc per milliliter to 900 μc per milliliter. To simplify calculations and measurements we obtain our supply from one source which ships a 10 mL ampule containing 2 mc. The decay factor can be determined from Table B-1. For any initial radioactivity, the radioactivity per milliliter on a given day may be calculated. For example, on day 3, the radioactivity of our preparation is 2 × 0.774 = 1.548 mc per 10 ml. An initial radioactivity of 2 mc per 10 ml is preferred because the volume used for stock solution preparation is at least 1 ml. Solutions of greater specific activity would entail using fractions of a millimeter. The "stock" solution is freshly prepared weekly by dilution of the original shipper's solution.

TABLE B-1. Decay Factor

Days	Factor
1	0.918
2	0.843
3	0.774
4	0.711
5	0.653
6	0.600
7	0.551
8	0.506
9	0.465
10	0.427

PREPARATION OF "STOCK" SOLUTION. The stock solution is used for injection into patients and for the preparation of standards. Since syringes pre-calibrated for delivery are used, a 5 ml volume is preferred for injection. To obtain a dose of about 15 μc for a 5 ml injection approximately 150 μc I^{131} HSA is diluted with normal saline solution in a 50 ml stock bottle. If the original shipper's solution contained 200 μc per milliliter, a 1 ml portion is diluted. If the original solution contains more or less radioactivity, that quantity containing 150 μc can be calculated as follows:

$$\text{Volume} = \frac{150\ \mu c}{\mu c \text{ per ml} \times \text{decay factor}}$$

Thus on the third day with a shipping slip assay of 200 μc per milliliter,

$$\text{Volume} = \frac{150\ \mu c}{200 \times 0.774}\ 0.97\ \text{ml}$$

Since the measurement of blood volume is a dilution procedure, the exact number of microcuries per milliliter is relatively unimportant except to allow for the injection of a safe, adequate dose. In the example above, 1 ml would be used for dilution.

Under aseptic conditions, 1 ml (more or less) of original solution is aspirated into a syringe and injected into a rubber-capped sterile ampule containing 50 ml of isotonic saline solution in distilled water containing preservative.* This is the stock solution containing about 3 μc per milliliter. Syringes pre-calibrated to deliver 5 ml, 7 ml, and 10 ml are available to allow for decay so that nearly 15 μc are injected in a single dose. After preparation of standards, the stock solution is stored in a lead container under refrigeration.

PREPARATION OF STANDARDS. The standard solutions are prepared from the stock solution on the same day the latter is prepared from the original shipper's solution. Approximately 8 ml of stock solution is aspirated into a clear, dry test tube. Two milliliters of *accurately* pipetted aliquots using the same pipette are quantitatively transferred to each of three 1000 ml volumetric flasks half filled with approximately normal saline solution (2 level teaspoons NaCl per liter of tap water) and mixed by swirling. In all accurate pipette transfers, standardized pipettes should be used. These are critical measurements. Care should be taken to wipe the outside of the pipette before adjusting the fluid to the 2 ml mark since an extra 0.1 ml introduced into the dilution flask will cause a 5 percent error. The inherent errors of the I^{131} human serum albumin method are less than 5 percent (124, 270). The flasks are filled to the mark with normal saline solution and mixed by inversion 20 times. Two milliliters of aliquots from each of the three standards is accurately pipetted into a clean, dry counting tube. Each tube is counted for about 10,000 counts in a scintillation well

---

*Commercial houses do not prepare 50 ml ampules. We stock 30 ml ampules of normal saline solution with preservative to fill our 50 ml sterile ampules.

counter. If the count rate varies by more than 1 percent, new standards are used as long as the stock solution is used for injection.

The rate of decay in the standard and in the stock solution used for injection is the same. The strength of the stock solution is easily calculated from the decay table. This calculation is necessary to inject a volume containing approximately 15 μc. The *exact* volume of stock solution injected into the patient must be known because this volume diluted in count value by the patient's blood is compared with the count in a *known* volume of stock solution diluted to a known volume with normal saline solution. It is apparent that for any tagged dilution procedure

$$V_1 \times C_1 = V_2 \times C_2$$

where

V_1 = volume of tracer substance

C_1 = concentration of tracer in solution

V_2 = volume of diluted tracer

C_2 = concentration of diluted tracer

PROCEDURE ON THE PATIENT. Syringes, pre-calibrated for delivery, are used for injection. The volume of solution injected includes the volume in the barrel of the syringe, the needle hub, and the needle bore. Twenty-two gauge 1-1/2 inch needles are used; 5 ml and 10 ml syringes allow a range of 5 ml, 7 ml, and 10 ml pre-calibrated volumes. The usual volume of 5 ml stock solution is injected into the vein of one arm and rinsed once with blood. Ten minutes later (although less time is needed) approximately 8 ml of blood is drawn from a vein in the other arm and transferred to a heparinized test tube. The tube is stoppered and mixed gently by tipping it up and down. If the patient has had any recent administration of isotopes, a control heparinized blood is drawn before the injection of stock solution. The syringe number and the volume of solution injected are recorded.

COUNTING PROCEDURE. Similar volumes (2 ml) of standard, whole blood, and plasma are accurately pipetted into clean, dry counting tubes. After the samples of whole blood or of whole blood and control blood are transferred, the plasma is separated by centrifugation at 2500 rpm for 10 minutes. The room background count (*BG c/s*) is measured.

The time for 100 registers is measured. One register = 64 counts, so that the time for 6400 counts is recorded. The counts per second are derived from:

$$c/s = \frac{6400}{\text{time (seconds)}}$$

The isotope blood volume (*IBV*) or plasma volume (*IPV*) is obtained from

$$IBV \text{ or } IPV = \frac{(c/s \text{ std})}{(c/s \text{ vol}) - (BG)}$$

$$\times \text{ dilution factor} \times \text{ volume injected}$$

The correction for previous isotope administration is as follows:

IBV or *IPV*

$$= \frac{(c/s \text{ std}) - (c/s \text{ }BG)}{(c/s \text{ vol} - c/sBG) - (c/s \text{ control vol} - c/s \text{ }BG)}$$

No one substance measures blood volume. From the ratio of counts in unit volumes of plasma label injected and plasma after mixing one obtains the *measured* plasma volume *MPV*). An estimated blood volume (*EBV*) may be obtained from *MPV* by the formula

$$EBV = \frac{MPV}{(100 - CH)} \times 100$$

where *CH* represents the venous hematocrit corrected for trapped plasma (*vide infra*). Similarly, the dilution of labeled red cells in the total red cell mass will give the *measured* red cell volume (*MRCV*), and the estimated blood volume (*EBV*) may be obtained from the formula

$$EBV = \frac{MRCV}{CH} \times 100$$

The Corrected Venous Hematocrit (CH). It has been reported that plasma trapped in the red cell column of centrifuged blood may be as low as 2 percent (192) or as high as 8.5 percent (45). Variations in technique are blamed for these discrepancies. Leeson and Reeve (166) state that "all workers using hematocrit methods should state the anticoagulant used, the dimensions of hematocrit tubes, the lengths of the columns of blood in them, the radius of the centrifuge head, the speed and time of centrifugation and the correction factor applied." Using heparinized blood in a Wintrobe tube filled to the 100 mark and a routine clinical centrifuge at 3000 rpm with a 15 cm head (1500 × *g*) for 30 minutes, the correction factor 0.96 (230, 46) or 0.95 (166) may be used. If centrifugation time is lengthened to 55 minutes, the correction factor 0.975 (360) may be used. With the longer centrifugation time factors of sedimentation rate, abnormal cell size, and alteration in plasma viscosity play a lesser role. We use a 30-minute centrifugation time and the correction factor 0.96.

The Isotope Hematocrit (IH). An "isotope" hematocrit may be calculated from the radioactive count of the plasma tag in whole blood and in plasma. A count on whole blood and on an equal volume of plasma must relate directly to the dilution of plasma by cells. The limits of accuracy are determined by a volume measurement and the counting. Accuracy is independent of variables that affect the centrifuge hematocrit.

$$IH = \frac{BV - PV \times 100}{BV}$$

where BV is the volume of blood estimated from dilution of the isotope in whole blood and PV is the measured plasma volume from dilution of the isotope in plasma. A similar formula has been suggested by Zipf, Webber, and Grove (366);

$$IH = 100 \left(1 - \frac{S_B}{S_P} \right)$$

where S_B and S_P represent the specific activity of whole blood and plasma.

The isotope hematocrit is a direct measure of the venous hematocrit and agrees well with the corrected centrifuge hematocrit on venous blood (*CH*). In a large series of observations (215)

$$\frac{IH}{CH} = 1.0 \pm 0.03$$

While we in our laboratory routinely check the venous hematocrit, one may readily substitute *IH* for *CH* in the formula for estimating blood volume (Equations 1 and 2 below).

The Body Hematocrit (BH) and the BH/CH Ratio. It has been accepted for many years (98, 285) that the volume percentage of red blood cells is not the same in all parts of the circulatory system. The radio of red cells to plasma is smaller in small vessels and capillaries and larger in large vessels and red cell depots (e.g., spleen). True total measured blood volume (*MVB*) is the sum of the measured plasma volume (*MPV*) and the measured red cell volume (*MRCV*); i.e.,

$MVB = MPV + MRCV$ and the true

$$BH = \frac{MRCV}{MPV + MRCV}$$

It is practical to measure either plasma volume or red cell volume and *estimate* the whole blood volume from the measured volume and the corrected venous hematocrit (*CH*) according to the following formulas:

From measured plasma volume,

$$EBV = \frac{MPV}{100 - CH} \times 100 \qquad (1)$$

From measured red cell volume,

$$EBV = \frac{MRCV}{CH} \times 100 \qquad (2)$$

Equations 1 and 2 will be correct only if *BH* equals *CH*. Since *BH* is lower than *CH*, *EBV* from Equation 1 overestimates *MBV*, and *EBV* from Equation 2 underestimates *MBV* by about 10 percent. If the relationship of *BH* to *CH* is fairly constant, a correction factor can be applied to the *EBV* formula. In normal humans and in many disease states the average *BH/CH* ratio is 0.91 (19, 26, 27, 46, 105, 208, 248). The estimated blood volume formula changes as follows:

From plasma volume,

$$EBV = \frac{MPV}{(100 - CH \times 0.91)} \qquad (3)$$

From red cell volume,

$$EBV = \frac{MPV \times 100}{(CH \times 0.91)} \qquad (4)$$

The value for the *BH/CH* ratio depends upon accuracy in cell and plasma volume measurements. In rats it has been found to vary from 0.98 to 0.74 (130, 237). The accuracy of the technique may be questioned, as has been done with similar reported variations in humans (215). The relative constancy of the *BH/CH* ratio through wide variations in venous hematocrit level has been demonstrated by Chaplin, Mollison, and Vetter (47). Further accurate simultaneous determinations of measured red cell and plasma volumes are needed in various pathological states to establish the range of the *BH/CH* ratio. It is possible that conventional methods of estimating blood volume may not be applicable in all clinical conditions. There is little doubt that the method is of value in normal humans and in many with disturbed functioning.

MEASUREMENT OF RED CELL VOLUME

The most commonly used isotopes for tagging red blood cells are P^{32}, Cr^{51}, Fe^{55}, and Fe^{59}. In 1950 Sterling and Gray (296) introduced radioactive sodium chromate ($Na_2Cr^{51}O_4$) as a red cell tag. Because of many advantages, the Cr^{51} method has virtually replaced all other isotope methods for labeling red blood cells. In vivo synthesis is unnecessary, it does not injure red cells (360), it allows lower radiation levels (217), and liquid counting can be done in a well-type scintillation counter. A disadvantage is that labeled cells are unstable if stored for over 24 hours in normal saline solution, for Cr^{51} is lost from cells and sequestration of cells occurs soon after injection.

Radioactive sodium chromate ($Na_2Cr^{51}O_4$) is a pure gamma emitter and has a half-life of 27.8 days. Commercial preparations have a specific activity of about 1.5 mc per milligram, and the usual dose of 50 μc contains approximately 0.3 mg of chromium. Chromium binds to hemoglobin and is eluted at a constant rate of 1 percent per day (217). When the chromated cell is destroyed, the chromium does not label other cells. Since there is so little loss after injection, the post-injection sample can be taken at a convenient time. The addition of ascorbic acid to a mixture of blood and sodium chromate ($Na_2Cr^{51}O_4$) reduces the anionic hexavalent form to the cationic trivalent form, which does not penetrate red cells but is capable of labeling plasma proteins. While it is not essential to wash the cells before injection, it is necessary to correct for cationic chromium in the plasma. The details of the technique as employed in our laboratory are as follows:

PREPARATION OF "BOTTLE BLOOD." Thirty milliliters of venous blood are aspirated into a sterile 50 ml heparinized syringe. The blood is injected into a sterile 50 ml rubber-capped bottle containing about 10 ml ACD solution. Fifty to 75 μc CR^{51} as sodium chromate ($Na_2Cr^{51}O_4$) in approximately 1 ml are injected into the bottle. During 30 minutes' incubation at room temperature, the bottle is gently swirled several times. Fifty milligrams of ascorbic acid in about 1 ml of solution are injected into the bottle, reducing the chromium to cationic chromium and preventing further intracellular incorporation. This preparation is referred to as "bottle blood."

PATIENT PROCEDURE. Exactly 20 ml of well-mixed "bottle blood" are injected by pre-calibrated syringe into one of the patient's antecubital veins, and the syringe is rinsed once with the patient's blood. After a 15-minute mixing period, 10 ml of patient venous blood are drawn from a different antecubital vein, introduced into a clean, dry, heparinized test tube, and used as follows:

1. 2 ml are transferred to a clean, dry counting tube (IV).

2. 2 ml are used for venous hematocrit determinations (VI).

3. The remaining blood is centrifuged and 2 ml of plasma are transferred to a clean, dry counting tube (V).

PREPARATION OF STANDARD.

1. 2 ml of mixed "bottle blood" are transferred to a 1000 ml volumetric flask half filled with distilled water to which five drops of concentrated HCI have been added. The flask is filled with water and thoroughly mixed by inversion (20 times). Then 2 ml of this solution are transferred to a clean, dry counting tube (I).

2. 2 ml of mixed "bottle blood" are transferred to a hematocrit tube for "bottle hematocrit" determination (III).

3. The remaining "bottle blood" is centrifuged, and 2 ml of the supernatant are transferred to a 1000 ml volumetric flask containing distilled water. The flask is filled, the contents are mixed by inversion 20 times, and 2 ml of this solution are transferred to a clean, dry counting tube (II).

Counts are done on tubes I, II, IV, and V and corrected for background count. The following data are now available:

I—net *c/s* on 2 ml 1-500 diluted "bottle blood"

II—net *c/s* on 2 ml 1-500 diluted "bottle supernatant"

III—bottle hematocrit × 0.96

IV—net *c/s* on 2 ml patient blood

V—net *c/s* on 2 ml patient plasma

VI—patient venous hematocrit × 0.96 (*CH*)

The estimated blood volume (*EBV*) is obtained from Equation 5.

$$EBV = \left[\frac{(I)}{(IV)} - \frac{(100 - III)(II)}{(100 - VI(V)} \right]$$

$$\times 500 \times ml \text{ "bottle blood" injected} \quad (5)$$

The red cell volume (*RCV*) is obtained from Equation 6.

$$RCV = EBV \times CH \quad (6)$$

Correction for body hematocrit may be made from *EBV* (Equation 7) or *RCV* (equation 8).

$$BV = EBV \times \frac{CH}{CH \times 0.91} \text{ or } BV = (EBV)(1.10) \quad (7)$$

$$BV = \frac{RCV}{(CH)(0.91)} \times 100 \quad (8)$$

CORRELATION OF BLOOD VOLUME MEASUREMENT WITH BODY PARAMETERS

Isotope methods for measuring the plasma volume and red cell volume have been standardized and simplified to the point where they are readily employed in the routine clinical isotope laboratory. Numerous attempts have been made to correlate measurements with various body parameters such as weight alone (with or without correction factors), height and weight, surface area (11), lean body mass (22), and more recently the cube of height and total body mass (4). In addition, certain anthropometric parameters such as biacromial diameter and skin fold thickness have been suggested. Clinical expediency precludes the use of ideal conditions and complex parameters. Even if refined standard conditions of measurement were to yield predictable blood volumes, such conditions for measurement could seldom be duplicated in clinical practice.

With a choice of measurement of either the plasma volume or the red cell volume by methods detailed above, it seemed desirable to determine the blood volume in a group of normal human adults. Since the I^{131} labeled human serum albumin method is technically easier than the labeled red cell method, it was chosen for the measurement of plasma volume and estimation of the total circulating blood volume under controlled conditions. Only the simple parameters of sex, weight, and height were used. From these data it was hoped that correlation with simple body parameters could be obtained in the development of prediction formulas for circulating blood volume. Further, these data could be used to check on the accuracy of prediction formulas available in the literature.

The circulating blood volume of 155 normal adults was estimated using a factor for venous hematocrit (0.96) and body hematocrit (0.91). There were 92 men and 62 women with an age range of 17 to 90 years. Body weights ranged from 80 to 390 pounds, and heights ranged from 58 to 76 inches. An effort was made to avoid a biased population. None of the subjects gave a history of blood loss, anemia, rapid sedimentation rate, or debilitating or malignant disease.

The blood volumes obtained were plotted against three of the most commonly used formulas for predicting blood volume: (1) the body weight formula, (2) the surface area formula, and (3) height cubed–body mass formula. Since a direct ratio of measured to predicted blood volume is desirable, a 45-degree line passing through the origin is the only mathematically acceptable line of regression. If correlation is perfect, all points will fall on this regression line. The degree of correlation depends upon the extent to which the points on the plots cluster into an ellipsoid whose major axis approximates collinearity with the 45-degree slope, and upon the distribution of the points about the major axis (ratio of major to minor axes).

THE BODY WEIGHT FORMULA
(75 ML PER KILOGRAM TIMES BODY MASS)

The average normal circulating blood volume has been reported to be 75 ml per kilogram (110). Females have smaller blood volumes than males or an average of 66 ml per kilogram. The sex difference has been explained on the basis of greater mass of metabolically inactive fat tissue in relation to the total volume mass in females.

When measured blood volumes of our patients were plotted against the body weight as a sole parameter (Figure B-3), poor correlation, as evidenced by lack of ellipsoid clustering of the points and of collinearity with the 45-degree line, was obtained. In fact, large differences between actual blood volume and predicted blood volume were found. There seems no longer reasonable justification for retaining the body weight formula as a method of predicting circulating blood volume.

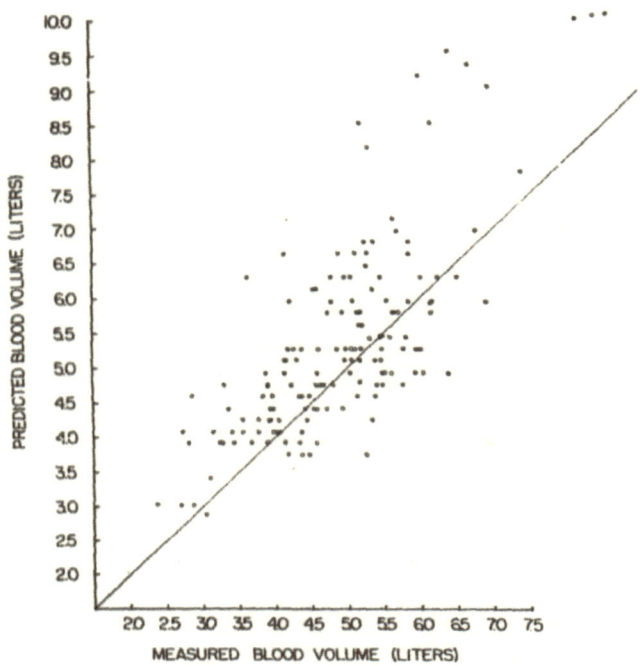

FIG. B-3. Measured blood volume (I^{131} human serum albumin): 75 ml per kilogram times body mass in kilograms. (Courtesy of C.V. Mosby Co. from "Prediction of blood volume in normal human adults." Nadler, S.B., Hidalgo, J., and Bloch, T., *Surgery 51*:224, 1962.)

THE SURFACE AREA FORMULA
(2.68 LITERS PER SQUARE METER TIMES SURFACE AREA)

This formula was proposed and used by Baker and his associates (11), in a study of 150 clinical subjects using I^{131} tagged human serum albumin for determining the plasma volume. Although they recognized the sex difference in volume, no attempt was made to separate men and women; there was no correction for body hematocrit. Figure B-4 shows our measured blood volumes plotted against the volume predicted by the surface area formula. The points form an ellipsoid of reasonable dimensions, but the major axis is obviously skew to the 45-degree slope regression line—an adequate objection to the acceptance of this formula. Statistical analysis indicates how this formula might be improved (215, 122).

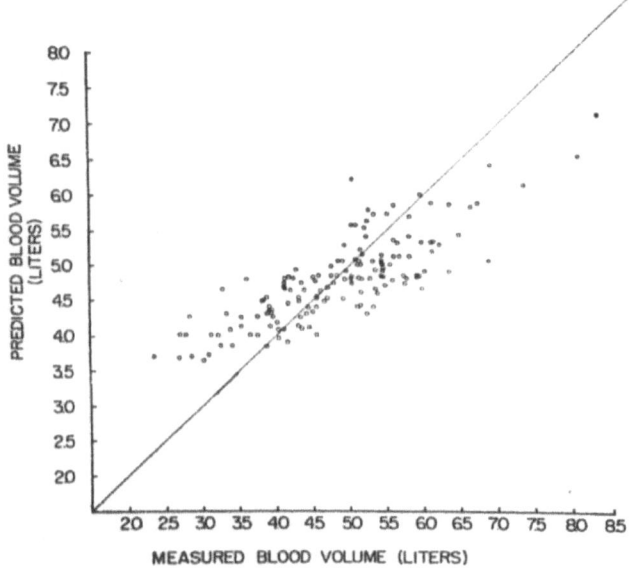

FIG. B-4. Measured blood volume (I^{131} human serum albumin): 2.68 liters per square meter times surface area in square meters. (Courtesy of C.V. Mosby Co. from "Prediction of blood volume in normal human adults." Nadler, S.B., Hidalgo, J., and Bloch, T., *Surgery 51*:224, 1962.)

THE HEIGHT CUBED–BODY MASS FORMULA

The major deviations from the mean using the body weight formula and the surface area formula can largely be attributed to differences in adiposity. Allen and his colleagues (4) studied Chinese subjects by densitometry and skin flow measurements to determine the lean body weight and applied their formula to the prediction of circulating blood volume. They used the T-1824 dye method for plasma volume measurement and appropriate corrections for "adiposity factor." Corrections for "trapped" plasma (0.96) and body hematocrit/venous hematocrit ratios (0.91) were used.

Figure B-5 shows our measured blood volumes plotted against the volumes predicted by the height cubed–body mass formula. While the major axis of the ellipsoid is more nearly collinear with the 45-degree slope regression line, the distribution about this axis is wider than with the surface area formula.

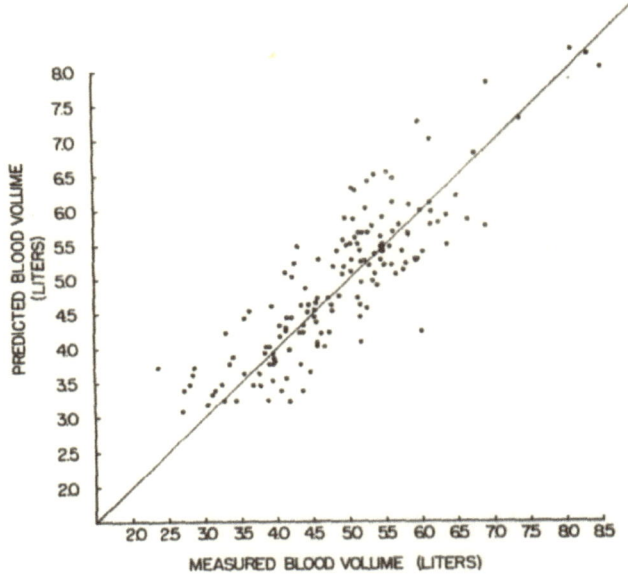

FIG. B-5. Measured blood volume (I^{131} human serum albumin): height cubed–body mass formula. (Courtesy of C.V. Mosby Co. from "Prediction of blood volume in normal human adults." Nadler, S.B., Hidalgo, J., and Bloch, T., *Surgery 51*:224, 1962.)

REGRESSION FORMULA

It seemed worthwhile to explore the potential of the IBM electronic digital computer in performing a regression analysis. The computer offered an opportunity to compare several formulas—a Herculean task by any other method. The equipment performs a series of approximations to minimize the sums of squares of deviation of the measured blood volume from the predicted blood volume. In essence, there is an automatic performance of the method of least squares. The program of Cates and his group (44) was used. The patients were separated into male and female groups and the surface area and height cubed–body mass formulas were examined by the computer method of regression analysis. The basic surface area formula is of the form

$$PBV = \alpha_1 H^{0.725} W^{0.425}$$

where *PBV* is predicted blood volume, α_1 is a constant, *H* is height (in centimeters) and *W* is weight (in kilograms).

Using this formula the computer indicated a value for α_1, and a correction factor yielding the following prediction formulas:

For men,

$$PBV = 0.0236 \times H^{0.725} \times W^{0.425} - 1.229 \qquad (9)$$

where 1.229 liter is the correction factor supplied by the computer to compensate for the skewness shown in Figure B-6.

For women,

$$PBV = 0.0248 \times H^{0.725} \times W^{0.425} - 1.954 \qquad (10)$$

Figure B-6 shows the distribution of data when the measured blood volumes of our men and women were plotted against the computer-corrected surface area formula. This formula shows the loss of skewness, and statistical improvement in correlation was also found (122).

The basic height cubed–body mass formula is of the form

$$PBV = \alpha_1 H^3 + \alpha_2 W + \alpha_0$$

where PBV is predicted blood volume, α_1, α_2, and α_0 are constants, H is height (in meters) and W is body mass (in kilograms).

Regression analysis gave the following formulas:

For men,

$$PBV = 0.03669H^3 + 0.03219W + 0.6041 \qquad (11)$$

For women,

$$PBV = 0.03561H^3 + 0.03308W + 0.1833 \qquad (12)$$

Figure B-7 shows the plot of measured blood volume of our males and females against volumes predicted by the computer-corrected height cubed–body mass formulas. While improvement over the uncorrected formulas is difficult to decide visually, statistical data indicated significant improvement in correlation (215).

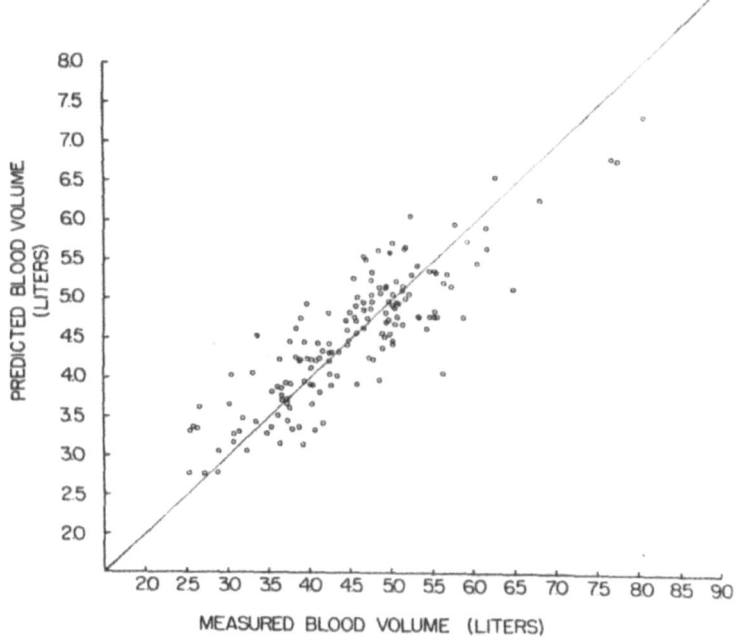

FIG. B-6. Measured blood volume (I^{131} human serum albumin): computer-corrected surface area formula. (Courtesy of C.V. Mosby Co. from "Prediction of blood volume in normal human adults." Nadler, S.B., Hidalgo, J., and Bloch, T., *Surgery 51*:224, 1962.)

On the basis of the statistical data, it was concluded that neither the *uncorrected* surface area formula nor the *uncorrected* height cubed–body mass formula fitted all populations. On the other hand, the computer modifications of the surface area formula and the height cubed–body mass formula fitted all populations equally well. It was not possible to distinguish statistically between the blood volumes predicted by the computer-corrected surface area formula and those predicted by the computer-correlated height cubed–body mass formula. Tables B-2 and B-3 give a schedule of predicted blood volumes based on height and weight for men and women.

A practical test of the validity of the prediction of the formula is obtained if plots of the measured blood volumes, done by different investigators using varied techniques, against the predicted blood volumes show good correlation. The measured blood volumes of 81 patients in Allen's series (4), and 82 cases of Gibson and Evans (97), both of whom used T-1824 dye to measure the plasma volume, were corrected for centrifuge hematocrit and body hematocrit factors and plotted against the computer-predicted blood volume. These data are shown in Figure B-8. Wennesland and his co-workers (345) used Cr^{51} to tag red cells of 201 males to measure the red cell volume. The measured red cell volumes with appropriate corrections for venous hematocrit and body hematocrit yielded "measured" blood volumes. These were plotted in Figure B-9 against computer-predicted blood volume. Figure B-10 is a composite plot of 518 measured blood volumes of normal adults using either plasma or red cell tag done by different investigators. These data indicate that the correlation is as good as might be expected from the method, regardless of whether red cell or plasma radioactive tag or dye tag is used, provided that corrections for centrifuge hematocrit and body hematocrit are made. The usefulness of the prediction formulas appears to be demonstrated.

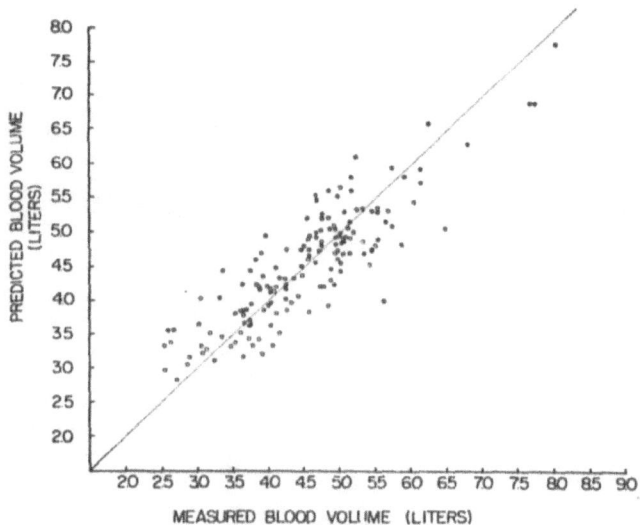

FIG. B-7. Measured blood volume (I^{131} human serum albumin): computer-corrected height cubed–body mass formula. (Courtesy of C.V. Mosby Co. from "Prediction of blood volume in normal human adults." Nadler, S.B., Hidalgo, J., and Bloch, T., *Surgery 51*:224, 1962.)

TABLE B-2. Predicted "Normal" Blood Volumes, Males

$$(PBV = 0.0236 \ H^{0.725} \ W^{0.425} - 1.229)$$

Height (in)

Weight (lb)	60	62	64	66	68	70	72	74
100	3342	3452	3561	3669	3776	3882	3988	4092
110	3531	3645	3759	3871	3983	4093	4203	4312
120	3710	3829	3947	4063	4179	4294	4408	4521
130	3881	4004	4126	4247	4366	4485	4603	4720
140	4044	4171	4297	4422	4545	4668	4790	4910
150	4201	4332	4461	4590	4717	4844	4969	5093
160	4352	4487	4620	4752	4883	5012	5141	5269
170	4498	4636	4772	4908	5042	5175	5307	5439
180	4639	4780	4920	5059	5196	5333	5468	5603
190	4775	4920	5063	5205	5346	5485	5624	5761
200	4908	5055	5202	5347	5491	5633	5775	5915
210	5036	5187	5336	5484	5631	5777	5922	6065
220	5161	5315	5467	5619	5768	5917	6064	6211
230	5283	5440	5595	5749	5902	6053	6204	6353
240	5402	5562	5720	5877	6032	6186	6339	6491
250	5518	5680	5841	6001	6159	6316	6472	6626
260	5632	5797	5960	6122	6283	6443	6601	6758
270	5743	5910	6076	6241	6405	6567	6728	6887
280	5851	6021	6190	6358	6524	6688	6852	7014
290	5957	6130	6302	6472	6640	6807	6973	7138
300	6062	6237	6411	6583	6754	6924	7092	7259
310	6164	6342	6518	6693	6866	7038	7209	7378

TABLE B-3. Predicted "Normal" Blood Volumes, Females

$$(PBV = 0.0248\ H^{0.725}\ W^{0.425} - 1.954)$$

Height (in)

Weight (lb)	60	62	64	66	68	70	72	74
80	2414	2520	2624	2727	2829	2931	3032	3132
90	2639	2749	2859	2967	3075	3182	3288	3393
100	2849	2965	3079	3193	3305	3417	3528	3638
110	3048	3168	3287	3406	3523	3639	3755	3869
120	3236	3361	3485	3607	3729	3850	3970	4089
130	3416	3545	3673	3800	3926	4051	4175	4298
140	3588	3721	3853	3984	4114	4243	4371	4498
150	3752	3890	4026	4161	4295	4427	4559	4690
160	3911	4052	4192	4331	4468	4605	4740	4874
170	4064	4209	4353	4495	4636	4776	4915	5053
180	4212	4361	4508	4653	4798	4941	5084	5225
190	4356	4507	4658	4807	4955	5102	5247	5392
200	4495	4650	4804	4956	5107	5257	5406	5554
210	4630	4788	4945	5101	5255	5408	5560	5711
220	4761	4923	5083	5242	5399	5555	5710	5864
230	4889	5054	5217	5379	5539	5699	5857	6013
240	5014	5182	5348	5513	5676	5838	5999	6159
250	5136	5307	5476	5644	5810	5975	6138	6301
260	5255	5429	5601	5771	5940	6108	6274	6439
270	5372	5548	5723	5896	6068	6238	6407	6575
280	5486	5665	5843	6018	6193	6366	6538	6708
290	5598	5780	5960	6138	6315	6491	6665	6838

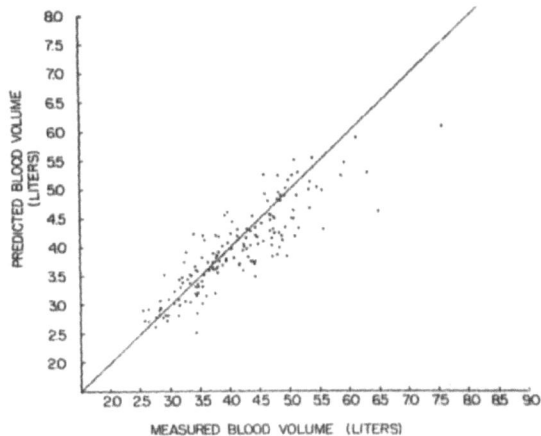

FIG. B-8. Measured blood volume (T-1824 method): computer-predicted blood volume. (Courtesy of C.V. Mosby Co. from "Prediction of blood volume in normal human adults." Nadler, S.B., Hidalgo, J., and Bloch, T., *Surgery 51*:224, 1962).

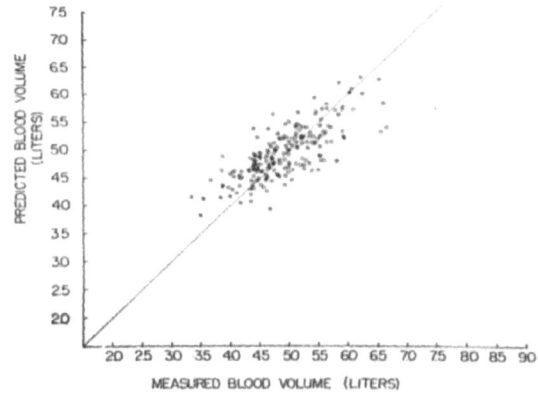

FIG. B-9. Measured blood volume (Cr[51] method): computer-predicted blood volume. (Courtesy of C.V. Mosby Co. from "Prediction of blood volume in normal human adults." Nadler, S.B., Hidalgo, J., and Bloch, T., *Surgery 51*:224, 1962).

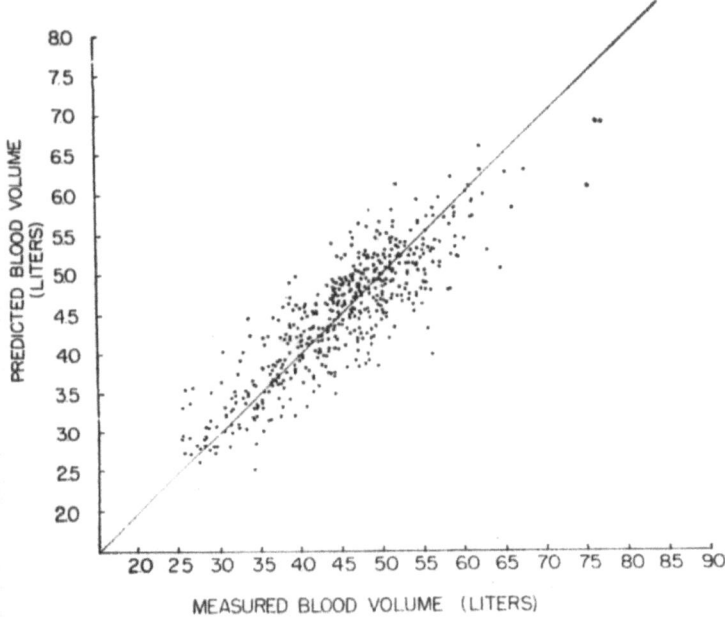

FIG. B-10. Measured normal adult blood volumes (518 cases): computer-predicted blood volume. (Courtesy of C.V. Mosby Co. from "Prediction of blood volume in normal human adults." Nadler, S.B., Hidalgo, J., and Bloch, T., *Surgery 51*:224, 1962.

Gunnar Sevelius, MD

APPENDIX C
REGIONAL BLOOD VOLUME
MEASUREMENTS

Gunnar Sevelius & Steve Creekmore

STEWART'S EQUATION defining the mean transit time as being

$$\frac{\text{Volume}}{\text{Volumetric flow rate}}$$

may be used to determine volume, provided independent methods for estimating mean transit time can be found. It can be shown that mean transit time corresponds to the difference between the times of centroids of dye dilution curves taken from the input and output of any fluid reservoir. When the indicator is injected instantaneously into the input, the centroid for the outflow curve is necessary. This method is the classical method for determination of regional volumes (297).

PULMONARY VOLUME
Dock *et al.* (73) and Milnor *et al.* (207) injected nonradioactive tracer simultaneously into the pulmonary artery and the left atrium and sampled from a peripheral artery. The difference in centroid times of the two recorded time concentration curves yields the pulmonary volume.

Dock's mean value for normals was 246 ml/m^2 surface area. For patients with valvular disease but without heart failure, Milnor *et al.* found a range for pulmonary volume of 126-598 ml/m^2 surface area, with a mean of 365 ml/m^2 surface area. These two studies are the best estimates of pulmonary volume and may be used as references.

Making use of the centroid of the right and left heart in the radiocardiograph, Lammerant (158, 161) estimated the volumes of left heart and lung to be a mean of 689 ± 128 ml/m^2 surface area and found a significant correlation between this estimate and the central blood volume determined according to Hamilton (115).

Approximations of centroid time have been introduced to avoid the laborious procedure for determination of centroid. Pietila and Hakkila (235) used the time difference between peaks of the right and left heart in the radiocardiogram. In a radiocardiogram the peak of the left heart is shifted because the left heart curve is added to the downslope of the right heart curve. Therefore, it is necessary to separate the right and left heart

115

curves before measuring the difference between the peak times. In our mathematical model it was found that the peak time corresponded closely to the residence time in lung and left heart, if the lung flow characteristics can be assumed to be essentially constant from individual to individual. Pietila found a correlation coefficient of 0.9 with the arm-to-arm volume. His values were in the range of Dock and Milnor with a mean of 300 ml/m^2 surface area.

The basic differential flow equation (Equation 42, Appendix A) offers a possibility to calculate the pulmonary volume if one can assume perfect mixing in each chamber system and rodlike flow through the lungs. The recorded count rate of the right heart (R_{rh}) is then proportional to the concentration and volume:

$$R_{rh} = \alpha_{rh} C_{rh} V_{rh} \tag{1}$$

This yields a record of the concentration of material entering the lungs. If the left heart is likewise perfectly mixed, the differential equation for left heart may be written

$$V \frac{dC_{lh}}{d\theta} = F(C_i - C_{lh}) \tag{2}$$

where C_{lh} is related to R as before:

$$R_{lh} = \alpha_{lh} C_{lh} V_{lh} \tag{3}$$

At the maximum of the left heart curve

$$\frac{dC_{lh}}{d\theta} = 0 \tag{4}$$

and therefore, here

$$C_{i\ lung} = C_{lh} \tag{5}$$

The curve for the outflow of the lung is identical to the curve for the right heart, because of rodlike flow, delayed in time by the average residence time. The average residence time, λ_{ave}, through the lungs is the time difference between the left heart peak and the downslope of the right heart at the same height (Figure C-1). The left heart peak height should be corrected for its geometry. This can be done by comparing R_{max} for each side of the heart, after they are corrected for dilution by a function of their respective θ'.

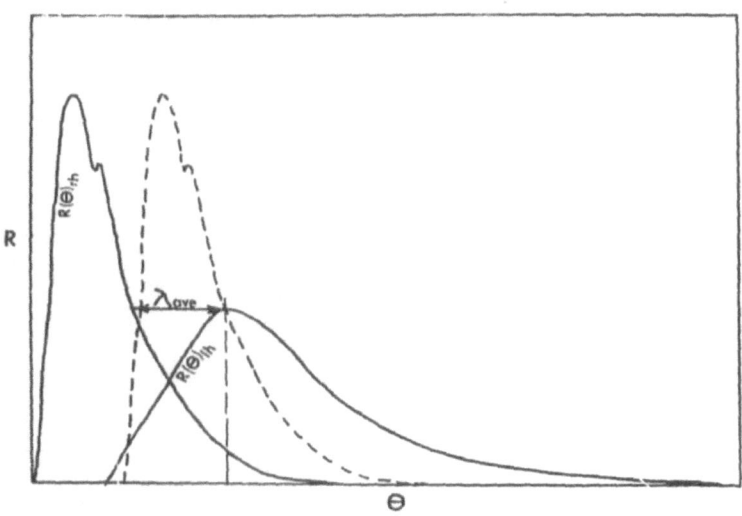

FIG. C-1. Illustration of method for determining λ_{ave} assuming equal geometric factors.

The pulmonary volume (V_P) is thereafter calculated as

$$V_P = \lambda_{ave}CO \qquad (6)$$

Pulmonary volume as calculated by this technique has a mean of 292 ml/m$_2$ which agrees with the results of Dock and Milnor.

In Table C-1 we have determined the pulmonary volume in 11 patients according to the methods of Lammerant, Pietila, and the one proposed above.

The methods of Lammerant and Pietila yielded similar results, both a pulmonary volume of about 16% of the total blood volume. Our technique gave a pulmonary volume of about 10-11% of total blood volume. The difference of 4-5% would correspond to the volume of one side of the heart (221, 222). Both Lammerant and Pietila originally assumed that the left heart volume was included in their pulmonary volume.

Donato *et al.* (75, 76) injected radioactive tracer into the pulmonary artery and approximated the residence time of the lungs by taking the average of the shortest passage time and the time to the left heart peak, assuming that there is an equal distribution of transit times and that the longest transmit time corresponds to the time from injection to the left

TABLE C-1. Comparison of Methods of Lammerant, Pietila, and Powers

| Num-ber | Pulmonary Blood Volume | | | Pulmonary Blood Volume/M² | | | Pulmonary Blood Volume × 100/Blood Volume | | |
	Lam-merant	Pietila	Powers	Lam-merant	Pietila	Powers	Lam-merant	Pietila	Powers
666	761	666	452	413	362	245	15.7	13.6	9.2
757	1047	942	663	526	473	333	19.5	17.5	12.3
938	718	684	387	412	393	222	15.8	15.0	8.5
1140	997	881	592	486	429	289	18.0	15.9	10.7
1029	711	655	417	416	383	243	15.9	14.6	9.4
1155	915	864	617	440	415	297	16.6	15.7	11.2
1449	906	813	573	529	475	335	20.3	18.2	12.8
1263	929	947	643	474	483	328	17.7	18.0	12.2
1105	961	877	589	528	482	324	20.0	18.3	12.2
446	730	816	597	410	458	335	15.7	17.5	12.8
756	774	755	503	396	387	258	14.8	14.4	9.6
$\bar{M}$	859	809	548	457	431	292	17.27	16.24	10.99

heart peak. The values for pulmonary and left ventricle volume by this technique were within 211-403 ml/m² surface area, with a normal value of 312 ± 56 ml/m². All of the above described methods are based on assumptions. The truth will be known when the work of Milnor *et al.* is repeated together with radiocardiography.

PROPORTIONAL SCANNING

Another possibility for determining regional blood volume is offered by proportional scanning (274). After the tracer is homogeneously mixed with the blood, the thoracic blood pool volume (V_t) is determined by doing a whole body count with (cts_2) and without (cts_1) the thorax region shielded. The thoracic blood pool volume is then

$$V_t = \left(\frac{cts_1 - cts_2}{cts_1} \right) BV \qquad (7)$$

where BV is the total blood volume. The critical assumptions here are that the absorption and geometric factors are the same for all blood in the body. The former seems reasonable, and the latter can be achieved by placing the scanner a long way from the body. Since the angle subtended by the body is small, the geometrical orientations of different body parts are nearly the same. We placed the person lying on his let side with his back to the crystal and oriented him along an isodose line, 7 feet from the crystal. Using this technique, we found that the thoracic blood volume was about

41 percent, the head volume 6 percent, and the volume of the lower legs about 10 percent of the total blood volume.

HEART VOLUME

Whole-heart volume can be measured using x-ray techniques such as those described by Nylin. Two x-rays are taken to get perpendicular cross-sectional representations of the heart. If the heart can be considered to be ellipsoidal and symmetric in the planes of the x-rays, then the displacement volume is simply

$$V = \frac{\pi}{6} d_1 d_2 d_3 \quad (d_1 d_2 d_3 \text{ are the axes of the ellipse}) \quad (8)$$

Since exact measurement of the three diameters is sometimes difficult, one of the equivalent formulas

$$V = \frac{2}{3} Af d_3 \tag{9}$$

or

$$V = \frac{8}{3\pi} \frac{Af A}{h} \tag{10}$$

(A = saggital area. Af = frontal area. h = common height of Af and A.)

is sometimes used. It can be shown that if the x-ray viewing planes are not parallel to the axial planes of the ellipse, then the calculated volume will be larger than the actual volume (221, 222). Equation 10, then, appears to be a better approximation (Nylin). The method has certain drawbacks. The heart outline must be clearly visible on the x-ray. The distention of the pericardium alone may give a false impression of heart enlargement. Also, of course, the heart is not exactly ellipsoidal in shape. Nylin did achieve a close correlation between heart volume measured by x-ray and actual heart displacement determined by post mortem examination. According to Nylin, the volume of the heart by x-ray is one-third larger than the actual blood volume in the heart.

A diagnostic problem often difficult to settle is that of an enlarged heart on account of a pericardial effusion. Different advanced techniques with help of x-ray fluoroscopy have been advocated, but none seem to always be able to establish a conclusive diagnosis. Many times the question has to be settled by pericardial puncture. Together with x-ray the problems can now be solved by blood pool scanning as described in

Appendix F. An alternative solution for those who do not have a scanner available will be proposed here.

The technique is based on the formula

$$\left[(cpm)_{heart} \div \left(\frac{cpm}{ml} \right)_{blood\ sample} \right] k = ml_{heart\ blood\ pool} \quad (11)$$

The detector is placed over the heart silhouette as suggested by a chest x-ray. The count rate is recorded, a blood sample is withdrawn, and the concentration of radioactivity in the whole blood is determined in a well counter.

In order to calculate the volume of blood under the counter according to Equation 11, it is first necessary to perform the procedure on a patient whose heart volume is known, for instance from a 2 plane chest x-ray, as suggested by Nylin. The equation may then be solved for the geometric factor k. When the geometric factor is once established for the system, it may be used in subsequent determinations (275).

A similar technique was reported at the same time by Love and Burch (181, 229). Their calculations were based on the same mathematical formula, but they used collimation of the detector.

HEART CHAMBER VOLUME

Right chamber volume may be estimated if an injection is made instantly into the right ventricle and complete mixing can be assumed to take place immediately (75, 76). The clearance slope from the right side will then be dependent on the cardiac output and the volume of right ventricle according to the equation

$$R(t) = R_p \exp\left(-\frac{Ft}{V} \right) \quad (12)$$

where R_p is the peak height and t is the time to the peak height. The stroke volume is easily calculated rom the cardiac output. The residual volume in the right ventricle may then also be determined. The assumption of complete mixing of the bolus with the blood in the right chamber when the bolus is injected directly into it should be taken with some reservation.

The radiocardiogram can be used to estimate the monitored volume of each side of the heart by the formula:

$$V_M = \frac{COA}{R_{max}} \qquad (13)$$

R_{max} should be corrected for dilution with a function of θ'. The estimate is actually on the monitored volume of each side of the heart. This can be made very close to the actual volume by proper collimation. Of the techniques proposed here for determining heart volume, this method is the simplest and probably the most accurate.

CORONARY VOLUME

As the geometry for the coronary bed is approximately the same as for the two sides of the heart, the volume of the coronary bed can be calculated very simply from the relationship

$$V_c = \frac{A_c V_{(R+L)}}{A_{(R+L)}} \qquad (14)$$

This measurement may prove to be very important in evaluating arteriosclerotic heart disease. Theoretically, one can expect that a widespread arteriosclerotic process has a small flow was well as a small coronary volume. On the other hand, a localized arteriosclerotic process will have a small flow but normal volume.

Acknowledgement

The authors wish to express their thanks to Mrs. Clare Patterson for her technical assistance and for preparation of illustrations.

Gunnar Sevelius, MD

APPENDIX D
CARDIAC OUTPUT

Gunnar Sevelius

THE CLASSIC METHOD for the determination of cardiac output is based on the Fick (88) principle, now almost a hundred years old. This makes use of a clearance speed in order to calculate the cardiac output. The arteriovenous concentration difference of a gas is determined while the total amount of tracer gas cleared is controlled. The arteriovenous concentration difference divided into the amount of tracer cleared per unit time yields the blood flow.

THE RUBIDIUM[86] TECHNIQUE

Love and Burch (177, 179, 182) used the Fick principle for determination of cardiac output in dogs, using the radioactive tracer rubidium[86]. During a continuous infusion of the tracer into the pulmonary artery, the arterial concentration was determined by means of an arterial puncture and the venous concentration by sampling the pulmonary artery proximal to the infusion. The cardiac output (F) was calculated as

$$F = \frac{Rb^{86} \text{ uptake}}{Rb^{86} \text{ A - V difference}}$$

(Rb^{86} uptake = Rb^{86} injected – Rb^{86} in the blood – Rb^{86} in the lungs.)

The Rb^{86} in the lungs was determined in autopsy material from the dog. During this explorative work the investigators found that the arterial concentration of the Rb^{86} correlated with the cardiac output as determined by a dye dilution technique. The correlation suggested that the uptake speed of the substance in the lungs as reflected in the arterial concentration could be related to the cardiac output and might be used as a clinical test. The regression line of the equation for this correlation also suggested the plasma space between the injection and the sampling. Since only an arterial sampling was necessary for the determination of cardiac output, this method may prove simple enough for clinical use. Ten microcuries of Rb^{86} was necessary during a five-minute infusion period. A correlation coefficient of 0.97 with the dye technique was established with a mean error of less than 10 percent. The technique required an infusion pump and a regular well counter as equipment. The result was received from a single determination, rather than a complicated calculation including an extrapolation, as in the Stewart-Hamilton technique. The proposed simplified method can be compared to evaluating blood flow of an organ by measuring its oxygen uptake.

USE OF THE RADIOCARDIOGRAPH

In 1945 Prinzmetal (241) showed that a radioactive tracer substance in the blood stream could be monitored on the chest wall in a so-called radiocardiograph. Veal (53, 321, 322) and Huff (132, 133, 134) took up this idea and worked out a formula by which the radiocardiograph could be used for calculation of cardiac output. The surface counting technique eliminated arterial sampling. This technique appears to be an optimal alternative for the determination of cardiac output. It is so fast and simple for the patient and the doctor that from this standpoint it can be compared to the procedure of recording an electrocardiogram.

Veal's and Huff's formula for cardiac output may be written

$$F = \frac{E}{A} \times BV$$

where E is the equilibrium recording, A is the integrated area under the time-activity curve, and BV is the blood volume of the patient. Calibration is done automatically with the determination of the radioactivity in a blood sample taken at the same time that the equilibrium is recorded. Huff (132, 133, 134) introduced the expression "blood volume per minute" in order to describe the formula physiologically. The bolus size per minute shown in the integrated area when calibrated by the equilibrium reading may be expressed in milliliters per minute when multiplied by a blood volume factor. In Chapter 1 it is shown how the formula is mathematically derived and how the different vectors of flow influence the recordings.

The radiographic formula for cardiac output is correct if the monitored volume in the equilibrium recording is equal to the monitored volume in the time-activity curve. The monitored volume, which is a part of the radiograph, cannot be controlled from the surface. The equilibrium recording must be made at the same site on the body as the time-activity curve, with the patient in unchanged position and in the same metabolic state between the two recordings. All the aforementioned factors affect the blood pool under the counter. During an exercise test it is best to prime the blood with a small dose of tracer so that changes in monitored volume can be followed.

The detector may also be designed so that the uncontrolled factor of monitored volume will have as little influence as possible. This result is best achieved by keeping the monitored volume small by collimation. The problem has to be met by maintaining the sensitivity of the detector so that the tracer substance does not get too large and expose the patient to unreasonable amounts of radioactivity. A collimation with a half-value angle of around 30 degrees is suggested by those who have investigated the question (235). The collimation may be achieved with either a one-bore collimator or a multichannel collimator. Less radioactivity is needed with the multichannel collimator. A comparison between cardiac output determined by arterial sampling and that determined by surface counting using the wafer collimator is reported in Table D-1.

The crystal used by earlier investigators had a diameter of 1 inch. There has been a tendency to increase the diameter of the crystal to 2 inches, which enhances the sensitivity and decreases the tracer amount. We use a 2-by-2 inch crystal.

TABLE D-1. Comparison Between Precordial and Arterial Determinations

Number	Precordial	Arterial	% Difference
1	8.44	8.89	−4.8
2	7.06	7.15	−1.2
3	8.35	8.05	+3.7
4	7.84	7.45	+5.2
5	6.09	5.76	+5.7
6	8.04	7.34	+9.5
7	10.20	9.20	+10.8
8	7.41	6.47	+14.5
	$\bar{X}$ 7.93	$\bar{X}$ 7.55	$\bar{X}$ +5.4

$r = .915+$
$p = < .01 > .001$

The crystal used by earlier investigators had a diameter of 1 inch. There has been a tendency to increase the diameter of the crystal to 2 inches, which enhances the sensitivity and decreases the tracer amount. We use a 2-by-2 inch crystal.

In an exercise test the author uses a small portable detector (Figure 5, Chapter 2).

The impulses from the detector are fed into a ratemeter. The ratemeter should be designed so that it has a fast enough time delay to follow the rapid change of events in the bloodstream. We use a time delay which can be adjusted to the pulse rate. By this means, curve irregularities caused by volume changes during systole and diastole will be abolished, and the curve will have a maximum smoothness with minimum time delay. If the interest of the investigator is concentrated on the instant stroke volume of the heart, this may be studied with a very short time delay. The time delay or resolving time of the ratemeter varies with different sensitivity levels. With low sensitivity the resolving time of the ratemeter will be longer and the time delay should be proportionately shortened. Our heart recordings are made at a sensitivity level of 300 K with a time delay of 0.50 seconds for a pulse rate of 50-70, 0.32 seconds for a pulse rate of 70-90, 0.22 seconds for a pulse rate of 90-120, and 0.11 seconds for a pulse rate above 120 beats per minute.

The ratemeter feeds the integrated impulses to a rectilinear ink recorder. This is the fastest and simplest way to record the time-activity curve. The width of the ink recorder may be either 4 or 8 inches. Some investigators record the impulses on tape and integrate them by hand. If one is interested in following in detail the time events of the curve, this is an accurate method because there is no time lag. The tape recorder, however, has a drawback in that it has a relatively long resolving time. If impulses appear very fast, the crowded impulses will be lost. The needle deflection will not be linear in respect to count rate. Special tape recorders avoiding this effect are available.

The detector of the heart channel may be placed anywhere on the body where a flow curve can be registered, and where the monitored volume for the time-activity curve is equal to that of the equilibrium reading. Many investigators have been under the impression that the time-activity curve must be recorded over an artery. The design of the first machinery reflected this idea, showing different ways of collimating down on the aorta or some other major artery. With the small monitored volume in an artery and the small amount of radioactivity in this artery at any one time, it is hardly possible to register a flow curve even if the detector, with the mentioned sensitivity, is placed right over the aorta. Shipley (280), who exchanged dye for a radioactive tracer in the Hamilton technique, learned this by experience when he had to use a spiral instead of a straight tube for continuous blood sampling. Except for the heart chambers, the detector will record the bolus mainly as it passes a capillary bed and not an artery. We place the detector over the middle of the heart silhouette as suggested by x-ray fluoroscopy. The site over the left ventricle has been recommended by MacIntyre because the recorded curve gives a long clearance slope which facilitates semilogarithmic extrapolation.

The tracer substance usually is radioiodinated serum albumin. The amount of tracer varies with the grade of collimation, size of crystal, sensitivity level of the ratemeter, and size of the subject. For our wafer collimator we use 10-15 μc. The volume injected should be kept small, preferably less than one-half milliliter, in order to receive a sharp contour of the flow curve. When such a small volume of tracer is used, the portion of the volume left in the needle after injection constitutes a significant percentage. We prefer to count the syringe before and after injection in order to estimate the percentage of the total volume injected.

The patient may be placed in front of the detector sitting, lying, or sanding. Theoretically, the best position would be standing, in which position the heart would be moved forward toward the detector and abdominal organs kept away from the detector. In order to have comparative values for every patient, we record everyone supine, with the detector over his chest.

An example of a recording from our laboratory using a technique which we prefer is given in Figure D-1. The time events are expressed from right to left. In the radiocardiograph, there is a fast rise of the curve as the bolus passes the right heart. After a valley, while the tracer transverses the lungs, there is a second peak as the radioisotope passes the left heart. The area under each peak is independent of dilution but dependent on the volume of each heart side, the flow through them, and their distance from the detector.

The otherwise exponential downslope of the clearance curve from the left heart may slow a portion of convexity. This convexity will be further discussed in Chapter 5. Depending on the speed of the clearance from the heart and the speed of filling of the coronary circulation, the summation of the downslope may shift between convex and concave. When about 60 to 70 percent of the downslope is traced, the recirculation appears and distorts the rest of the curve. If the recirculation appears higher up on downslope of the left heart, the detector is usually placed below the heart. The distorted portion of the curve has to be extrapolated. This extrapolation may be achieved by semilogarithmic plotting.

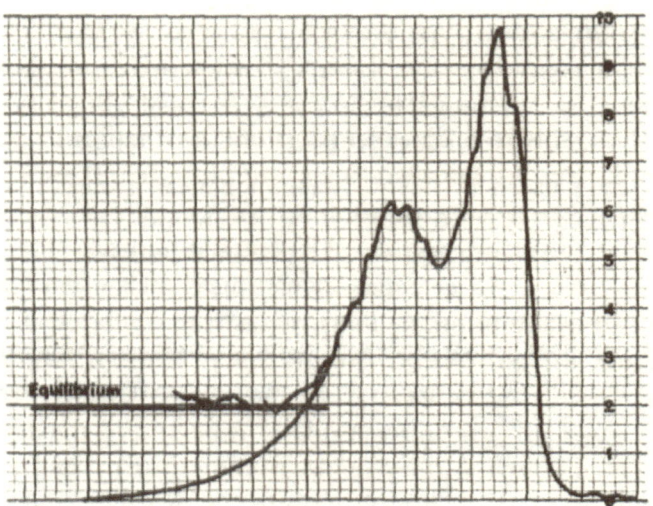

FIG. D-1. Example of a recording using author's preferred technique.

The area over the baseline and under right and left heart peak, and the coronary peak are measured with a planimeter. The equilibrium is measured with a ruler as the height between the baseline and the final recording after complete mixing.

The blood volume is determined by standards outlined in Chapter 4, and may be done as a separate procedure.

The cardiac output in liters per minute is received according to Veal and Huff's formula.

A person's cardiac output value is of no use if it cannot be judged against what should be normal for that person under the conditions in which it was determined. An attempt at such an evaluation is the cardiac index. Here the determined cardiac output value is corrected for the body size of the subject. However, many independent factors other than the size of the subject affect the cardiac output at a given moment. In different reports the cardiac index has a correlation coefficient with the determined cardiac output in normals of between 0.35 and 0.68. In our laboratory the correlation coefficient was 0.55 in a series of 700 determinations. Figure D-2 outlines the factors that control the cardiac output for a given person.

Cardiac Output

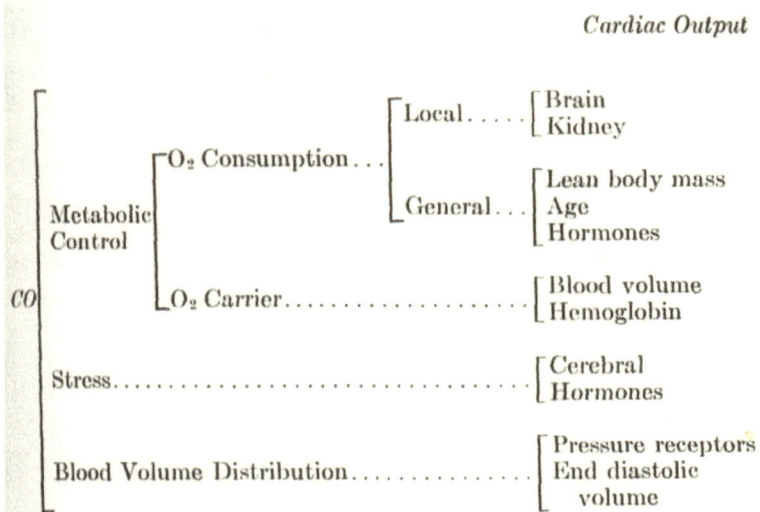

FIG. D-2. Outline of different factors that control cardiac output for a given person.

Under normal conditions the metabolic demand is determined by the lean body mass. This may be estimated from height and weight but should be modified by the age and sex of the person. The stress control may be checked by recording the pulse rate. The blood volume distribution should be considered normal for an estimated cardiac output. By correlating cardiac output in normal patients with the size, age, and pulse rate of each one we arrived at a regression formula for an estimated cardiac output. It is recommended that each laboratory establish its own regression formula as the collimation will affect the results slightly.

The estimated cardiac output in our laboratory has a correlation coefficient of 0.79 when compared with the actual determined cardiac output in normals. Comparing the actual with the estimated cardiac output enables one to make an informative clinical evaluation of the heart functions.

Gunnar Sevelius, MD

APPENDIX E
CORONARY BLOOD FLOW

Gunnar Sevelius

A TEST FOR SUCH A COMMON DISEASE as coronary arteriosclerosis must fulfill certain criteria in order to be of practical value in clinical medicine. It must be rapid and simple to perform. It must be relatively atraumatic so that it does not interfere with the care of these very vulnerable patients with coronary artery disease. The electrocardiogram fulfills these criteria, and no one will dispute its value in the diagnosis of coronary arteriosclerosis. However, the electrocardiogram records the disease process in the coronary artery indirectly by showing damage to the myocardium. The arteriosclerotic process in the arteries almost has to occlude the arteries before the electrocardiogram registers changes. The gradual pathologic changes before the final event cannot be detected by this means. It is likely that in the near future surgical, and possibly also medical, means will be introduced for diagnosis and therapy of coronary arteriosclerosis. For such treatment to be effective the arteriosclerotic process has to be diagnosed before the myocardium is damaged.

Because of its clinical significance, it is challenging to attempt to measure blood flow in general, and coronary blood flow in particular, with radioisotopes and surface counting. Since it was proved (289) that the coronary blood flow could be registered on the body surface, several different techniques have been tried for its determination. They may be grouped in three categories: (1) tissue saturation clearance or uptake, (2) tissue desaturation clearance, (3) volume clearance or tracer dilution. Terms applying to all techniques will first be pointed out. In surface counting, in general, a reading is dependent on two unrelated variables: one, the amount of radioisotope under the detector, the other, the geometry or percentage of total radiation emitted from the isotope that the detector actually registers. One cannot speak about a measured amount before geometry is defined. Other problems, specifically related to surface counting in the heart region, are the different volumes and the different tissues. If a volume clearance technique is tried the different flow curves from each volume have to be separated. If a tissue clearance technique is tried one should separate the clearance in the different tissues as well as volumes, particularly if the tracer substance does not have a preference for the tissue of interest. The monitored volumes in the heart region are so large compared to monitored tissue that a conservative and safe stand would be to consider any clearance recorded over the heart region as representing blood clearance in the chambers until proved otherwise.

In experimental work with dogs, total coronary blood flow can be determined by miniaturized electromagnetic flowmeters with great accuracy (276). In this kind of work there is no need for radioisotope methods. In clinical work, however, the need for a method measuring coronary blood flow is urgent.

The only earlier method of determination of coronary blood flow clinically is the nitrous oxide method, which determines the blood flow per 100 gm of left heart tissue. This technique, originally developed by Kety (147, 148) for the determination of brain flow, was adopted for the determination of coronary blood flow by Bing (27). It is based on the Fick principle or estimation of the blood flow from a clearance speed. The partition coefficient for nitrous oxide when it passes from tissue to blood or vice versa is first established. Once this is found and proved constant under different conditions, the clearance speed of nitrous oxide from the tissue can be related to blood flow per 100 gm of vital tissue. The clearance speed is calculated by determining the arterial and venous concentration of the tracer gas in multiple blood samples during the diffusion period. The blood sampling is done from the coronary sinus and an artery. The arterial puncture, and particularly the coronary sinus catheterization, at once limits the clinical value of the procedure.

Radioisotopes were introduced into the field of coronary blood flow determination through the nitrous oxide technique by substituting radioactive krypton for the nitrous oxide gas (165). This simplified the analysis of the samples, but because the catheterization is still necessary, no major steps toward wider clinical application have been taken. Other freely diffusible substances are apt to be tried. Before being accepted each new substance should be checked for eventual drug action on the coronary flow.

An interesting approach for the determination of any regional blood flow, including coronary blood flow, was introduced by Sapirstein (261). Potassium ion dissolved in the serum will immediately be absorbed intracellularly into vital tissue anywhere in the body. After an intravenous injection of potassium^{42} this ion divides between different organs in the same ratio as the bloodstream and is absorbed in each organ in proportion to the blood supply to the organ. Sacrificing the animal a given short time after the injection and determining the amount of potassium^{42} in each organ will yield the percentage of cardiac output that entered the organ. The potassium^{42} is a 20 percent gamma-ray emitter and has a half-life of 12.4 hours, which at the present time limits a wider use of this tracer.

Love and Burch (177, 179) had the intracellular uptake of potassium in mind when they introduced rubidium^{86} as a tool for determining regional blood flow. Rubidium is similar in physiological behavior to potassium. It is also an intracellular ion and is incorporated intracellularly very rapidly. It is a 20 percent gamma-ray emitter and has a half-life of 19.4 days, which makes it more suitable for laboratory work than potassium^{42}. Its diffusion into the heart muscle could be related to the blood flow by the Fick principle determining the arteriovenous difference or the diffusion process by surface counting over the heart and calculated an index of coronary blood flow by an empirical multiple regression formula. With the use of proper shielding, but otherwise not defined geometry, 70 percent of the counts could be estimated to come from the heart muscle. Mack and associates (189), following the rubidium uptake in isolated rabbit hearts, found that it was related not only to blood flow but to potassium concentration in the heart muscle. Gubner (111) pointed out that potassium is a very unstable ion in ischemic heart muscle. With many variables affecting the results, precaution must be taken in the interpretation. A hopeful improvement for the procedure has been introduced recently with rubidium^{84} (Bing, personal communication). This isotope is a positron emitter and discharges two gamma rays in opposite directions. With a detector placed over the heart, one on the anterior chest wall, and one on the posterior chest wall, and both detectors connected with a coincident circuit, the update can be limited to a funnel just between the two crystals. This technique will yield maximum uptake with minimum lead collimation. It will also yield a more fixed geometric pattern.

MEASUREMENT BY RADIOCARDIOGRAPHY

Waser and Hunzinger (339, 340) made use of the old established fact (Stewart 300, 301, 302, 303) that the coronary circulation was the first recirculation. They compared two total radiocardiographs, one with the total injected dose and one with the dose returning from the coronary circulation. The size of each radiocardiograph would be proportional to each dose and therefore would compare with the volumetric flow through the heart and the coronary. Although the theory is correct it has proved difficult to outline, particularly the radiocardiograph due only to coronary recirculation.

Together with Dr. P.C. Johnson, the author (272) started to record radiographs over the kidney region and the heart region simultaneously and found that as radioactivity entered the kidney region a convexity appeared on the otherwise supposedly concave exponential downslope of the peak from the left heart. This suggested that the peripheral circulation in the heart region was recorded in the radiocardiograph. Working with our surgical department we both occluded and separately perfused the coronary circulation while the tracer bolus passed through the heart (289). The curves suggested that the convexity seen with the coronary open consisted almost exclusively of coronary circulation on its first passage through the coronary bed.

Among the peripheral organs in the body the coronary bed has the advantage of being in a position such that its geometric factors are approximately equal to those of the heart. Once the flow curves are separated in the radiocardiograph, the geometric pattern of the coronary can be defined and blood flow calculated.

The technical requirements for determining coronary blood flow by radiocardiograph are the same as those used for determination of cardiac output. One may emphasize the importance of placing the detector close over the heart silhouette. The coronary blood flow as reflected in the radiocardiograph starts at the same time as other peripheral circulation. Only over the heart, and with proper collimation, does the peripheral circulation represent coronary blood flow.

LEFT HEART TRACING VS. ARTERIAL CURVE

In the radiocardiograph, Mena and his associates compared the downslope of the left heart, which is slowed by the coronary filling, with that of an arterially sampled curve. The closer to the heart the arterial curve is sampled, the more accurately the coronary delay can be determined. The downslope of the left heart, however, is dependent on the relative geometry of each chamber, the transit time in the lungs, and the coronary volume. All these factors are independent of coronary flow and the arterial curve which is used for comparison. The arterial sampling has to be done by blood sampling and not, as suggested, by surface counting; otherwise variable such as the monitored volume and geometry in the "arterial" curve will influence the calculations. The downslope of the left heart curve as compared to the downslope of the arterial curve was used as in index of coronary blood flow.

SCALING

Our own first endeavor to separate the coronary area from the left heart area was based on scaling alone (271). Analysis of the reproducibility suggested that we did not control all variables. Mathematical analysis of the flow led to the recognition of Z. The equation defining Z opened the door to a new approach. With the inclusion of the Z factor in the scaling procedure, we take this opportunity to present a technique for the interpretation of the radiocardiograph.

Cardiac output and monitored volumes of each side of the heart are first determined according to procedures outlined in Appendices B and A, respectively. The coronary area is separated from the left heart area by the Z curve for the left heart. The procedure of constructing a Z curve involves the following steps:

1. Calculate the Z number for the downslope according to Equation 49 in Appendix A.

2. Construct a vertical line at the point where the upslope intersects the baseline (Figure E-2).

3. On this line mark off the following heights: 5 percent, 20 percent, 50 percent, and 80 percent of the peak height.

4. Using the calculated Z factor for the one side of the heart, obtain the fraction $\dfrac{\theta}{\theta'}$ for each of the percent heights from Figure E-1.

5. Multiple each fraction by θ' to obtain the θ for each height.

6. Measure from the vertical line and mark the θ's at their respective heights.

7. Using the four resulting points, draw in the downslope of the heart curve. When the areas for the right and left heart and coronary are separated, coronary flow can be calculated.

In calculating the coronary blood flow, complete mixing in the left heart and rodlike flow in the coronary bed are assumed. Under these assumptions the input and output functions of the coronary bed are equal. The flow curve of the left heart will represent the input function of the coronary bed as there is no diluting volume between the two monitored volumes.

According to the basic differential flow equation we have for the coronary flow

$$\frac{dR_c}{d\theta} = \alpha_c F_c (C_i - C_o)_c \qquad (1)$$

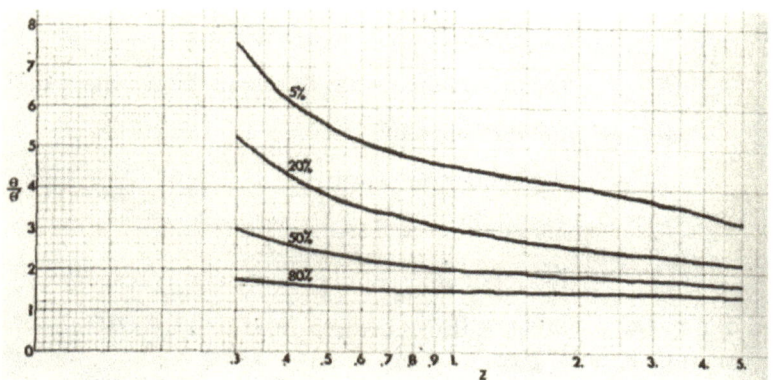

FIG. E-1. *Z* Chart.

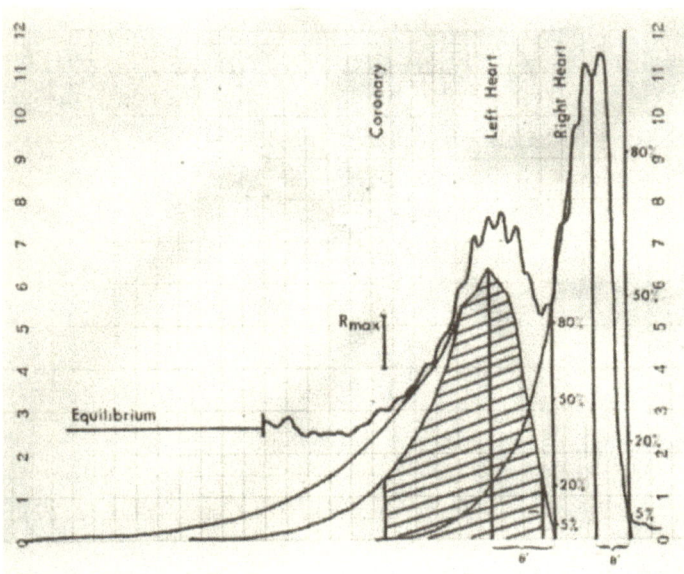

**FIG. E-2. Radiocardiogram separated in its
three main flow curves by scaling and *Z* factor.**

where

dR_c = the instantaneous count rate in the coronary bed

$d\theta$ = the time increment

α_c = the geometric factor

F_c = the volumetric flow rate

C_i and C_o = the input and output concentrations respectively

Integration of the differential flow equation from θ to 0 to $\theta = \theta'$ where θ' represents time to peak gives

$$\int_{R=0}^{R=R_{max}} dR = \int_{\theta=0}^{\theta=\theta'} \alpha_c F_c (C_i - C_o) d\theta \qquad (2)$$

$$R_{max} - 0 = \alpha_c F_c \int_{\theta=0}^{\theta=\theta'} \left[C_i(\theta) - C_o(\theta) \right] d\theta \qquad (3)$$

By rearrangement

$$\alpha_c F_c = \frac{R_{max}}{\int_0^{\theta'} C_i(\theta) d\theta - \int_0^{\theta'} C_o(\theta) d\theta} \qquad (4)$$

From the basic flow equation we have

$$A_c = \left(\frac{\alpha I V}{F} \right) \qquad (5)$$

Rearranged we have

$$I_c = \left(\frac{AF}{\alpha V} \right)_c \qquad (6)$$

I_c may also be expressed

$$I_c = F_c \int_0^\infty C_i(\theta) d\theta \qquad (7)$$

Combining Equations 6 and 7 and solving for the geometric factor we have

$$\alpha_c = \frac{A_c}{V_c \int_0^\infty C_i(\theta) d\theta} \qquad (8)$$

Inserting this geometric factor into Equation 4 we have

$$\left(\frac{AF}{V \int_0^\infty C_i(\theta)d\theta} \right)_c = \frac{R_{max}}{\int_0^{\theta'} C_i(\theta)d\theta - \int_0^{\theta'} C_o(\theta)d\theta} \quad (9)$$

By arrangement we have

$$F_c = \frac{V_c R_{max} \int_0^\infty C_i(\theta)d\theta}{A_c \left[\int_0^{\theta'} C_i(\theta)d\theta - \int_0^{\theta'} C_o(\theta)d\theta \right]} \quad (10)$$

The geometric factors for coronary bed and heart chambers are approximately equal. Since we know from Appendix A that the areas then correspond to the monitored volumes, we can write

$$A_c = \frac{A_H V_C}{V_H} \quad (11)$$

where V stands for volume, A for area, and subscript H for total heart. Substituting the expression for V_c of Equation 10 into Equation 9 and rearranging we have

$$F_c = \frac{V_H R_{max} \int_0^\infty C_i(\theta)d\theta}{A_H \left[\int_0^{\theta'} C_i(\theta)d\theta - \int_0^{\theta'} C_o(\theta)d\theta \right]} \quad (12)$$

As can be seen in Figure E-2,

$$\int_0^{\theta'} C_i(\theta)d\theta - \int_0^{\theta'} C_o(\theta)d\theta = \int_{0-\lambda}^{\theta'} C_i(\theta)d\theta \quad (13)$$

The integral $\int_0^{\theta'} C_i(\theta)d\theta$ is related to the actual count rate curve by the expression

$$\int_{0-\lambda}^{\theta'} C_i(\theta)d\theta = \frac{A'_{LH}}{\alpha_{LH} V_{LH}} \quad (14)$$

where A'_{LH} represents the cross-hatched area in Figure E-2.

139

In the same way the integral $\int_{0-\lambda}^{\theta'} C_i(\theta)d\theta$ is equal to $A_{LH}/\alpha_{LH}V_{LH}$, where A_{LH} represents the total area under the left heart curve.

Substitution of these expressions into Equation 10 gives

$$F_c = \frac{V_H A_{LH} R_{max} \alpha_{LH} V_{LH}}{A_H \alpha_{LH} V_{LH} A'_{LH}} \tag{15}$$

Therefore, finally we may calculate the coronary blood flow from

$$F_c = \frac{V_H A_{LH} R_{max}}{A_H A_{LH}} \tag{16}$$

Figure E-2 shows a radiocardiograph interpreted according to the outlined technique. The method was tested against electromagnetic flow meters for determination of coronary blood flow. The details of this study will be published elsewhere. The comparison was made in dog experiments with a collimator especially designed for the dog chest. The total range of difference was from −16 to +14 percent in 16 determinations with the mean difference being −8 percent. The comparisons were made in acute experiments where many variables such as the placement of the detector could be controlled. However, care should still be taken in extending the work to clinical evaluation. A 15 percent reproducibility can be accomplished by an experienced interpreter. The calculations are rather laborious and the author does not recommend use of the radiocardiograph without preceding practical instructions.

The radiocardiogram can now be separated into its three individual flow curves. It is within reason to believe that the one analysis of the radiocardiogram yields the total blood volume, the volume of blood in lungs, right heart, left heart, and coronary, as well as cardiac output, flow of blood in right heart, left heart, and coronary. The only trauma to the patient for this rather extensive information about his circulation is a venipuncture.

APPENDIX F

Reprinted from:

CLINICAL DYNAMIC FUNCTION STUDIES WITH RADIONUCLIDES

Editors:

Millard N. Croll

Luther W. Brady

H. Randolph Tatem III

Takashi Honda

Published by:

APPLETON-CENTURY-CROFTS

Educational Division

MEREDITH CORPORATION

440 Park Avenue South

New York, New York 10016

Gunnar Sevelius, MD

Short-Term Prediction of Myocardial Infarction or Sudden Death by Hemodynamic Assessment[*]

Gunnar G. Sevelius

PART I: Radiocardiogram and Its Clinical Assessment

Increasing public demand for preventive medicine has in recent years brought forward sophisticated hardware for mass screening. The lack of a specific test for a particular disease often justifies a multitude of tests for increased accuracy. Risk of heart attack, sudden death and stroke have been evaluated in this fashion.

Dangers, as well as blessings, from such predictive programs are proportional to the distribution of true and false, positive and negative results. A false positive prediction, marking the patient unjustly as a high risk, may well cause serious emotional and economic consequences. A false negative diagnosis, on the other hand, leads to false security at a time when preventive measures could be life saving.

In Part II of this report, the predictive value of cardiac output as a specific test in the short-term prediction of myocardial infarction will be discussed. The data and conclusions are based on serial hemodynamic measurements over a six-year period.

The determination of cardiac output in these studies was made by the radioisotope method, radiocardiogram. This technique lends itself well to screening purposes and follow-up examinations because it is quick, atraumatic, easily reproducible, and safe.[1]

The radiocardiogram is actually a time-activity curve recorded when the blood is followed with a radioactive tracer. The tracer substance is ^{131}I human serum albumin. The passage of the bolus through the heart is recorded by a scintillation detector.

With the patient supine, the scintillation detector is placed over the cardiac silhouette on the anterior chest wall. Following a 10-minute rest period for equilibration of the circulation, 10 to 15µCi of ^{131}I in less than

[*] This work was supported by the Federal Aviation Agency and the National Institute of Health, Grant HE 06946-07.

0.5 ml volume is injected rapidly into the antecubital vein. The 2 × 2 inch scintillation detector feeds into a ratemeter and a servorecorder (Figure F-1).

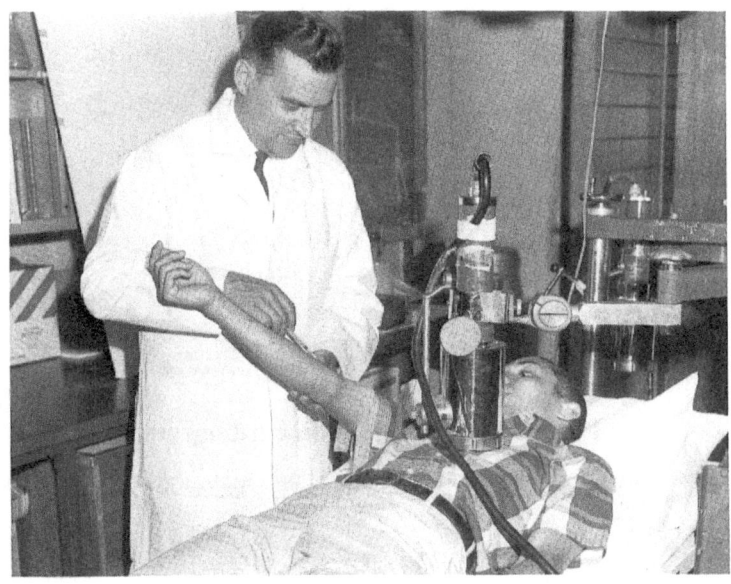

FIG. F-1. The procedure for recording a radiocardiogram.

Figure F-2 depicts a recording of a normal patient. The first rise of the curve is due to the bolus entering the monitored volume of the right heart. After a valley, during which time the tracer traverses the lungs, there is a second peak as the isotope passes the left heart. Depending on the speed of clearance from the left heart and the speed of filling of the coronary circulation, the configuration of the downslope may shift between convex and concave. When about 60% of the downslope is recorded, the recirculation effects distort the rest of the flow curve. The small distorted portion of the curve is easily computed by semilogarithmic extrapolation.

The area over the baseline, under the right and left heart, and the coronary peaks are measured with a planimeter. The equilibrium is measured with a ruler as the height between the baseline and a final recording after complete mixing. The blood volume is determined separately using ^{131}I human serum albumin. The procedure we prefer has been outlined by Nadler and Hidalgo[2], which uses ^{131}I human serum albumin in a standard dilution technique.

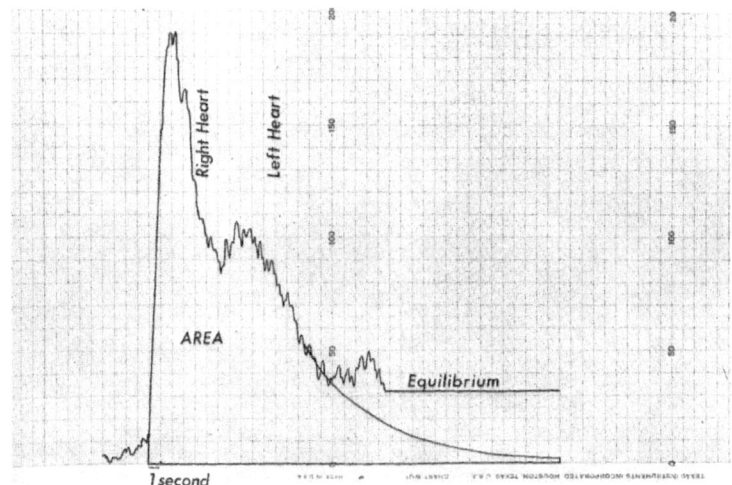

FIG. F-2. A sample radiocardiogram.

Cardiac output in liters per minute is calculated according to the formula:

$$F = \frac{E \times BV \times 3}{A} \qquad (1)$$

where F = cardiac output in liters per minute, E = equilibrium height in mm, BV = total blood volume in liters, 3 = conversion factor for the units in the formula, A = area under the time-activity curve in cm^2. The formula is self-calibrating because it expresses the ratio between two measurements, E:A, affected by the same variables such as sensitivity, amount of tracer dose, and monitored volume of traced blood. The effect that the blood volume has on the equilibrium, but not on the flow curve, is canceled by multiplying the equilibrium by the blood volume.[3] Basically, this formula, as well as the more commonly used Stewart and Fick formulas, can be derived from the basic flow concept: total amount of indicator = flow × the change in concentration of the indicator between the inflow and the outflow.[3] In the Fick formula, the change in concentration between inflow and outflow is the arterial-venous difference. In the Stewart formula and in formula (1) the change in concentration is expressed in the change of area of the dilution curve. The inflow area is zero because both formulas assume an instant injection into the inflow. Only the outflow area is therefore measured.

There is no significant difference between cardiac output measured by radiocardiogram and either Fick's or Stewart's methods.[411] We compared cardiac outputs by radiocardiogram and by Fick's and Stewart's methods in order to standardize our laboratory procedure. A high correlation was achieved following a few experiments. The results are listed in Figure F-3. There is no significant difference between the three techniques. The correlation coefficient was 0.9 with similar numerical values.

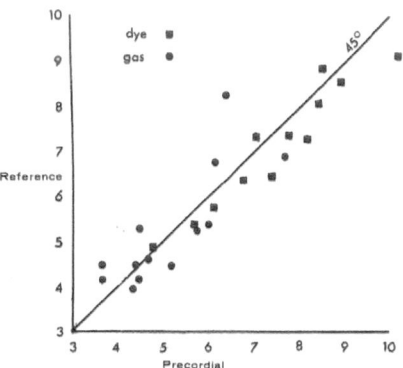

FIG. F-3. A comparison between cardiac output determined by radiocardiogram, Fick's gas clearance, and Stewart's dye dilution techniques. The units are in liters/min.

Figure F-4 correlates our numerical values with the values from eight different laboratories.

Cardiac output varies physiologically with sex, age, pulse, and blood volume.[12,17] An assessment must be made of each patient's determined cardiac output by comparing it to the cardiac output which is predicted from a normal subject of the same sex, age, pulse, and blood volume. The predicted normal value is computed by multiple regression formulas:

Male pred. CO = pulse × 0.0607 + BV × 1.67778 − age 0.05686 − 2.476

Female pred. CO = pulse × 0.0607 + BV × 1.67778 − age 0.02483 − 2.476

145

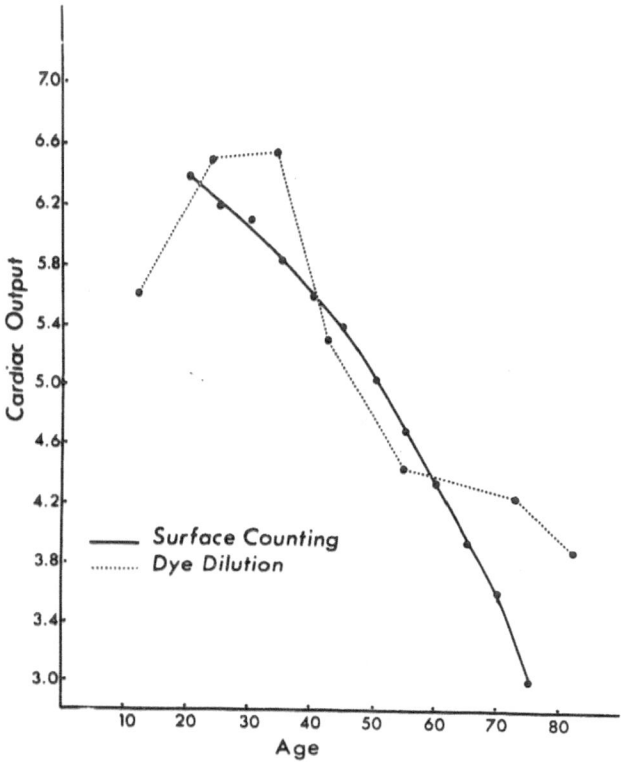

FIG. F-4. Age regression of cardiac output. The decrease in cardiac output by age as computed from the formula for prediction of cardiac output (solid line) and as determined by different investigators (dotted line). The dotted line represents a mean value as determined by eight independent laboratories. The values are marked in decades and the units are in liters/min.

The assessment will be referred to here as the "hemodynamic assessment" because it evaluates the relationship between the heart's function as a pump and the volume it has to pump. (Substituting body weight for body volume would yield a "metabolic assessment" of the cardiac output which might prove valuable in metabolic diseases.) The hemodynamic assessment is computed by the percent difference between the determined and the predicted cardiac output. The normal range for the hem0dynamic assessment is $100 \pm 20\%$.

Past clinical assessment of cardiac output has been based on the cardiac index which is obtained by dividing the cardiac output by the surface area of the patient. This corrects the cardiac output for a size-dependent variable, but leaves out the physiologic effect of pulse rate, blood volume, age, and sex.

The age regression according to our normal values is in Figure F-4, plotted against the mean cardiac output in different decades as reported in Table 34 of the National Research Council's Handbook of Circulation.[17] Both plots confirm that the cardiac output is only half at age 70 of what it normally is at age 20. This physiologic change can by itself account for the wide normal range (50% of the mean value) of the cardiac index listed from 18 studies in Table 35 in the same handbook. When the lower limit of a normal range is 2.3 (50%), and the upper limit is 5.0, it is very unlikely that the range can be used to detect early pathology. The physiologic change of the cardiac output due to age would also affect the normal range of stroke index.

Figure F-5 depicts graphically the last determined cardiac outputs from each control in our study. They are plotted against the hemodynamically predicted cardiac output in Figure F-5a and against surface area in Figure F-5b. The border of 95% confidence limit is marked with a dotted line. The regression line for cardiac index does not go through the origin. This is an absolute requirement if one wishes to normalize the cardiac output by simple division, as is done in the calculation of cardiac index. Tanner made the same observation and proposed a regression formula based on weight.[13]

Taylor and Tiede made a similar analysis and came to the same conclusion.[14] Smulyan et al. reviewed the world literature on cardiac index in a recent article[15] and proposed a multiple regression formula based on weight and height. They had a correlation coefficient of only 0.44 with the determined cardiac output.

The correlation coefficient for the results of our study in Figure F-4b (against surface area) was 0.45 (more than 0.5 is needed for significance). Blood volume, weight, and surface area have, in our experience, an identical correlation with the determined cardiac output.[16] The results of Sevelius and Modica were derived from a multiple regression analysis of 140 normal cardiac outputs and different physiological variables. The correlation coefficient for cardiac output and blood volume was 0.56671, surface area 0.56380, height 0.40981, and weight 0.56013. A high correlation could only be accomplished by correcting for age and pulse rate, together with a size-dependent variable. The correlation coefficient for the determined cardiac outputs and that predicted from blood volume, pulse, and age in Figure F-5a was 0.81.

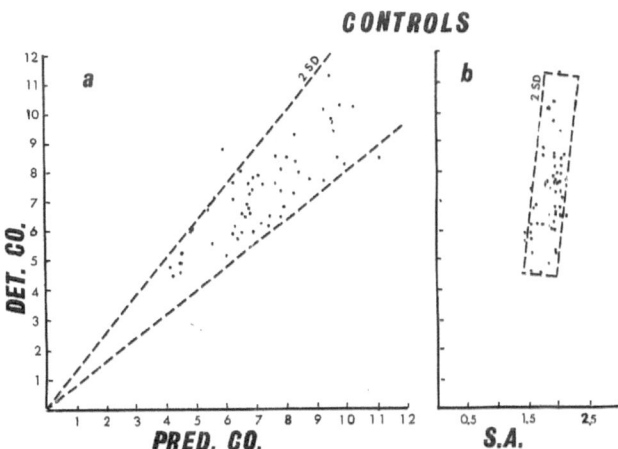

FIG. F-5. Comparison of determined cardiac output to a cardiac output computed from age, blood volume, and pulse (a) and also to surface area, (b) in controls. A 95% confidence limit is inserted with a dotted line. Units are in liters/min.

Our predicted normal values have been confirmed in controls from age 1 to 97 years. The male formula is common for both sexes before puberty, and after this females seem to age slower than do males.

The last cardiac output from each patient in our study is plotted in Figures F-6a and F-6b in the same way as Figure F-5. Results which proved to be true positive predictions are marked with triangles. The 95% confidence limit of the hemodynamic assessment depicts more than twice as many abnormal cardiac outputs as the cardiac index. A hemodynamic assessment always correlated with the clinical picture. The classification for functional capacity of the New York Heart Association may be translated into hemodynamic assessment in percent of normal, using 15% for each of its classes. Clinical signs of heart failure appear when the cardiac output has been below 70% for a significant period of time.

The indications for the determination of cardiac output reach into many fields of medicine. Any cardiovascular condition should be evaluated quantitatively so that medical treatment can be initiated before late clinical signs occur. Indications for cardiac surgery can more easily be assessed, and the difficult procedures objectively evaluated. Indications for cardiac output evaluation include elderly patients with limited cardiac reserve prior to major surgery, patients with severe, chronic fatigue, and those with metabolic disease.

An increase in blood volume makes the bloodstream "sluggish" in two ways: by straining the myocardium and by expanding the vascular bed. Renal diseases and drugs which affect fluid balance should be monitored, via the cardiac output assessment technique, for their possible affect on the heart. Any of these could lead to a high-risk state with a tendency toward intravascular thrombosis. Contraceptive drug side effects should also be monitored by this technique.

Hypertension is caused by changes in cardiac output, peripheral vascular resistance, changes in blood volume, or any combination of the three. A rational approach to therapy is accomplished by determining the underlying cause, and cardiac output assessment may be one of the more valuable adjuncts to diagnosis.

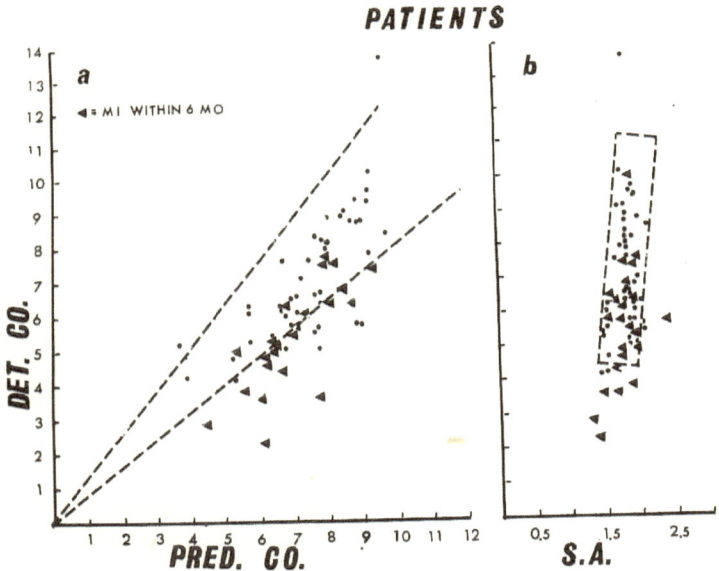

FIG. F-6. Comparison of determined cardiac output to predicted cardiac output (a) and also to surface areas (b) in patients. Triangles mark cardiac outputs measured within six months preceding a myocardial infarction or sudden death. Units are in liters/min.

Gunnar Sevelius, MD

Acknowledgement

The author wishes to express thanks to Professor A.C. Guyton for reviewing this report. Most of the credit for the completion of this lengthy study should go to the Chairman of the Department of Medicine, Dr. Stewart G. Wolf, who initiated development of methodology in 1957; his undivided support inspired an atmosphere of academic freedom and creativity.

Part II: Study Design and Results

The purpose of this study was to test the ability of cardiac output measurements to predict subsequent myocardial infarction or sudden death. Cardiac output has been measured shortly after myocardial infarctions and has usually been found to be low.[18-22] These low outputs could, of course, be the result of the infarctions, but it is also possible that low cardiac output preceded the myocardial infarctions and actually thromboses were precipitated by the slower blood flow.

PATIENT MATERIAL AND METHODS

The study subjects were followed from 1 to 72 months. The patient group consisted of 58 individuals of both sexes, varying in age from 30 to 84, who had recovered from a well-documented myocardial infarction a year or more prior to this study. The only exception was number 161, the youngest subject, who signed in as a control but developed an acute myocardial infarction during a treadmill test in the initial baseline workup. He was assigned patient status from then on. These subjects were studied together with 58 controls matched individually for sex, age, race, education, and occupation. Random selection was not complete, but bias was avoided by selecting patients from sequential admissions to the University Hospital and Veterans Administration Hospital. Controls were selected from a pool of more than 1,000 employees working for a highway department and two industrial firms in the vicinity. The selection of controls was based on the above criteria for matching and for geographical proximity to the study center. The criteria for the diagnosis of myocardial infarction were (a) typical clinical history and (b) unequivocal electrocardiographic and/or blood enzymatic changes. The admissions, the diagnosis, and all data were controlled by an expert executive committee from which the investigator and his associates were excluded. Fifteen different associates performed physiological, psychological, sociological, and dietetic evaluations. Detailed information on the design and content of the study has been reported elsewhere.[23] All measurements were, from the beginning, assessed for their predictive value since it was felt that such assessment would be the most objective way to gauge their relevance. Each patient subject was initially admitted to the hospital for one week, during which time baseline values were collected. Patient subjects were thereafter assigned to the care of a physician associate and were seen by him at six-week intervals. The investigator did not in any way participate in the care of the patients. Fifty-eight patients and 58 controls completed the flow measurement part of the study. Flow measurements were scheduled for each visit, which was many times during the first year. Later, only one, two, or three measurements were made per year. Not all subjects kept their appointments. On each visit the investigator determined cardiac output, blood volume, heart volume, and coronary blood flow. This report is concerned only with the results from the cardiac output measurements. Excluded from this report are nine individuals who started on the program but did not complete it. These consisted of one control and one patient who refused flow measurement determinations, one patient and one control from whom we were unable to obtain flow curves because of inability to puncture their veins, two patients who died of cancer, two patients who committed suicide, and one control who died of pneumonia.

The technique used for determining cardiac outputs and the calculations required to predict a normal value are discussed in Part I of this report. A clinical assessment of the subject, based on the amount his actual cardiac output deviates from his predicted normal value, is termed the "hemodynamic assessment." The normal range (2 SD) for cardiac outputs is $100 \pm 20\%$. A cardiac output of less than 80% of its predicted value leads to a hemodynamic assessment of high risk for a myocardial infarction in the ensuing six-month period.

RESULTS

A total of 669 cardiac outputs were determined during this study. The cardiac outputs in percent of their normal value are shown graphically in Figure F-7 for controls, in Figure F-8 for patients without subsequent myocardial infarction, and in Figure F-9 for both patients and controls with myocardial infarctions or sudden deaths while in the study. Fifty-seven controls without subsequent infarction had a total of 304 measurements ($\bar{x}$ = 5.2), and 31 patients without subsequent infarction completed 204 measurements ($\bar{x}$ = 6.5). Five patients and one control with nonfatal infarctions, and 22 patients with fatal infarctions or sudden death, had 160 measurements ($\bar{x}$ = 5.7). The longest observation period was 72 months; the shortest, one month; mean, 40 months.

In order to avoid overrepresentation, only the last curve from the controls (Table F-1) and from the patients without subsequent infarction (Table F-2) were compared to the last curve preceding an event in those who had myocardial infarctions or suffered sudden death within the six-month period following evaluation (Table F-3). The one control (072) who developed a myocardial infarction while in the study is listed in Table F-3. The risk of myocardial infarction or sudden death may be computed from the results depicted in these tables.

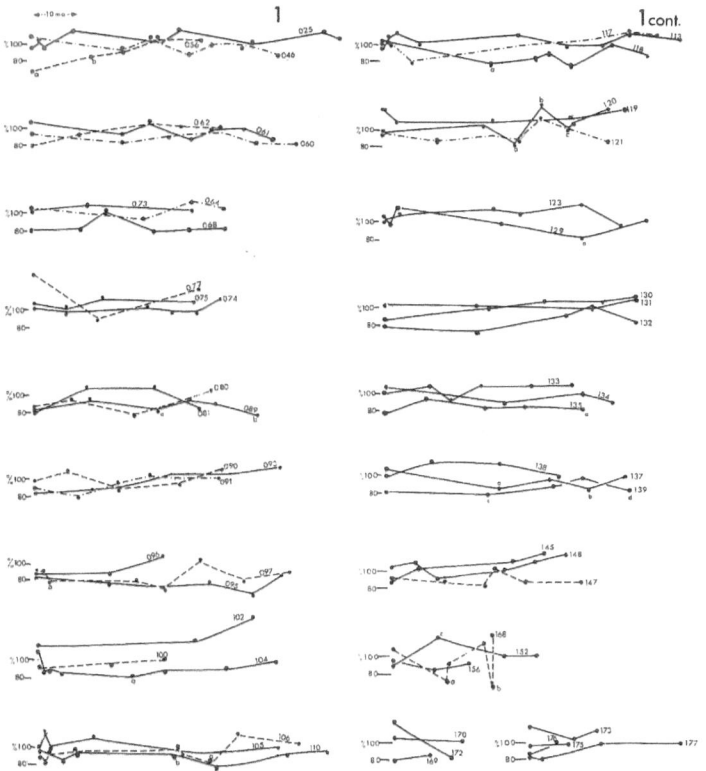

FIG. F-7. Hemodynamic assessment of control subjects: 046, emphysema; 095, emphysema; 106, (a) upper respiratory infection; 135, (a) nonspecific EKG changes; 137, (a) upper respiratory infection, (b) ACTH for acute arthritis; 147, emphysema; 168, (a) electrical conversion of fibrillation, (b) electrical conversion of fibrillation; 152, (c) "cold" and "coughing all night."

FIG. F-8. Hemodynamic assessment of patient subjects. No myocardial infarction or sudden death while in the study: 009, overweight (220 to 230 lbs., height 70 inches); 024, (a) diffuse T-wave changes, (b) digitalis started; 033, (a) leg and scalp lacerations in a train accident; 034, (a) upper respiratory infection; 041, emphysema, (b) "asthma acting up," (c) EKG loss of *Rv1* and *Rv2* but no clinical signs of myocardial infarction; 044, overweight (230 to 240 lbs., height 68 inches); 045, asthma and emphysema; 053, blood volume only 79 percent of normal; 066, (a) two days postprostatectomy, weak after operation, (b) angiogram shows right coronary artery occluded; 155, (a) recently digitalized; 153, (b) myocardial infarction two months prior to study while in exercise program; 161, (a) first myocardial infarction one week prior to study while performing treadmill test for admission to study.

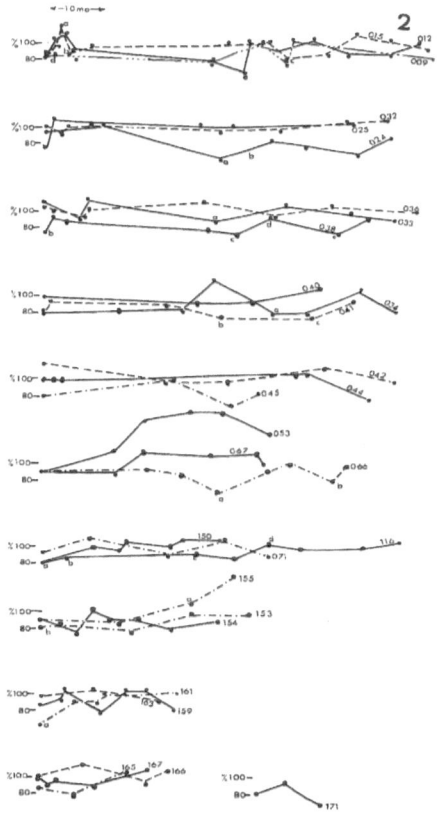

3

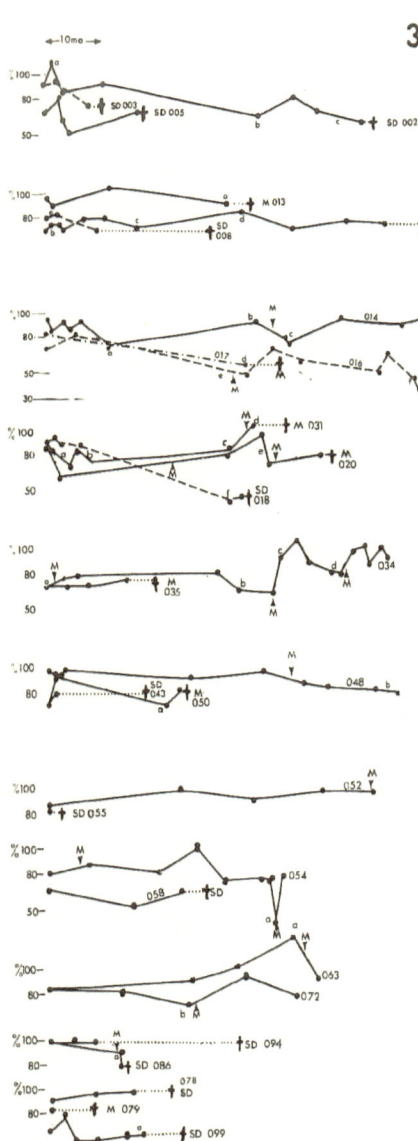

FIG. F-9. Hemodynamic assessment of patient subjects. Mycoardial infarction or sudden death while in the study: 003, (a) upper respiratory infection, fatal myocardial infarction while running to catch a bus; 014, (c) bigemini; 016, (e) pneumonia and myocardial infarction; 018, (f) dizzy, orthopnic; 054, (a) myocardial infarction on evening of day of assessment; 063, (a) alcoholically intoxicated at time of laboratory visit (less than six weeks after this visit a silent myocardial infarction); 072, (b) less than six weeks after this visit a silent myocardial infarction, EKG unchanged at the time; 086, (a) blood pressure before myocardial infarction 188/126 & 112/70 after, autopsy revealed hemorrhage in intima of left circumflex coronary artery; 078, sudden death in front of hospital after examination for chest pain, EKG one hour premortem unchanged, pain interpreted as peptic in origin, coronary blood flow during previous laboratory visit was 30% of normal; 099 (a) hospitalized for clinical heart failure.

TABLE F-1. Controls

N=57

ID	AGE	SEX	D	P	D/P	SA	CI	PRED.	COMMENTS
025	63	M	4.5	4.3	106	1.78	2.5	TN	
046	60	M	5.2	6.1	85	1.96	2.7	TN	
056	51	M	7.6	7.3	104	1.93	3.9	TN	
060	73	M	6.5	7.9	82	2.05	3.2	TN	
061	58	M	6.5	7.5	87	2.00	3.3	TN	
062	55	M	8.4	8.4	100	2.08	4.0	TN	
064	69	M	7.3	6.8	107	2.06	3.5	TN	
068	72	M	7.7	9.3	82	2.17	3.5	TN	
073	58	M	10.3	9.9	104	2.02	5.1	TN	
074	61	M	7.9	7.1	112	2.08	3.4	TN	
075	41	M	8.5	7.7	110	1.92	4.4	TN	
077	53	M	6.8	5.5	123	1.64	4.1	TN	
080	54	M	8.5	8.1	105	2.00	4.3	TN	
087	37	M	8.5	9.8	86	2.19	3.9	TN	
089	46	M	8.5	11.1	77	1.98	4.3	FP	
090	60	M	9.3	8.3	112	2.08	4.5	TN	
091	55	M	6.6	6.6	100	1.96	3.4	TN	
093	60	M	5.2	4.6	113	1.95	2.7	TN	
095	78	F	6.2	7.5	82	1.59	3.9	TN	Emphysema
096	72	F	8.5	8.0	107	1.80	4.7	TN	
097	72	F	5.7	6.5	88	1.55	3.7	TN	
100	46	M	7.6	7.7	98	2.04	3.7	TN	
102	62	M	8.8	6.0	147	1.80	4.9	TN	
104	47	F	5.9	6.3	94	1.54	3.8	TN	
105	72	M	6.5	6.7	97	2.19	3.0	TN	
106	58	F	6.9	6.8	102	1.67	4.1	TN	
110	77	F	7.4	7.9	93	1.58	4.7	TN	
113	59	M	7.4	6.9	108	1.86	4.0	TN	
117	60	M	7.6	6.8	112	2.00	3.8	TN	
118	41	M	7.8	8.9	88	2.06	3.8	TN	
119	35	M	11.3	9.5	119	2.10	5.4	TN	
120	64	M	6.0	4.9	123	1.95	3.1	TN	
121	61	M	7.3	8.3	87	2.04	3.7	TN	
123	61	M	6.2	6.4	97	1.79	3.5	TN	
129	46	M	8.1	7.9	102	1.95	4.2	TN	
130	49	M	7.8	7.0	111	1.98	3.9	TN	
131	47	M	10.1	9.3	109	1.90	5.3	TN	
132	53	F	6.2	7.2	86	1.70	3.6	TN	
133	82	M	4.9	4.5	110	1.91	2.6	TN	
134	57	M	6.3	7.1	90	1.98	3.2	TN	
135	63	F	6.5	8.0	81	1.88	3.5	TN	
137	60	F	5.6	5.6	100	1.53	3.7	TN	
138	76	F	4.6	4.6	100	1.59	2.9	TN	
139	65	F	5.2	6.1	85	1.63	3.2	TN	
145	63	M	6.1	5.0	122	1.86	3.3	TN	
147	67	M	6.0	7.0	85	1.96	3.1	TN	Emphysema
148	76	M	7.7	6.3	122	1.99	3.9	TN	
152	59	M	6.8	6.8	100	2.05	3.3	TN	
156	59	F	5.9	6.6	90	1.60	3.7	TN	

ID = *identification number*
D = *determined*
P = *predicted cardiac output in liters/min*
SA = *surface area of the body in m²*
CI = *cardiac index*
PRED = *prediction*
TN = *true negative*
FN = *false negative*
TP = *true positive*
FP = *false positive*

156

TABLE F-1. (continued)

168	73	M	7.1	5.6	126	2.06	3.4	TN
169	26	M	6.8	8.0	85	1.97	3.5	TN
170	36	M	9.7	9.6	101	2.00	4.9	TN
172	40	M	8.2	10.0	82	2.14	3.8	TN
173	69	F	4.8	4.2	114	1.49	3.2	TN
175	37	M	10.2	10.3	99	2.00	5.1	TN
176	31	M	6.7	6.9	98	1.75	3.8	TN
177	32	M	9.4	9.6	98	2.08	4.5	TN

TABLE F-2. Patients without Subsequent Infarction

N=31

ID	AGE	SEX	D	P	D/P	SA	CI	PRED.	COMMENTS
009	43	M	8.4	9.8	86	2.18	3.9	TN	
012	45	M	9.0	8.6	105	1.77	5.1	TN	
015	58	M	8.1	8.1	100	2.02	4.0	TN	
024	84	F	4.7	5.3	90	1.64	2.9	TN	
028	76	M	4.2	3.9	109	1.64	2.6	TN	
032	69	M	7.6	6.8	112	1.93	3.9	TN	
033	64	M	6.5	7.0	93	1.85	3.5	TN	
036	64	M	6.0	5.8	103	1.95	3.1	TN	
038	59	F	7.5	8.0	94	1.69	4.4	TN	
039	56	F	6.0	7.2	83	1.58	3.8	TN	
040	71	F	6.2	5.8	107	1.64	3.8	TN	
041	72	M	6.1	6.7	92	1.96	3.1	TN	
042	54	M	7.6	7.5	101	1.93	3.9	TN	
044	60	M	6.3	7.8	81	2.10	3.0	TN	
045	62	M	7.8	9.3	84	1.93	4.0	TN	Emphysema
053	83	M	5.1	3.7	138	1.93	2.6	TN	
066	59	M	7.0	7.3	96	2.06	3.4	TN	
067	66	M	6.8	6.8	100	1.97	3.5	TN	
071	61	M	6.5	7.2	90	1.93	3.4	TN	
116	56	M	9.3	8.9	105	1.96	4.7	TN	
150	43	M	8.8	8.1	109	1.92	4.6	TN	
153	42	M	8.7	8.8	99	2.07	4.2	TN	
154	59	F	5.2	5.8	89	1.53	3.4	TN	
155	45	M	13.6	9.7	140	1.90	7.2	TN	
159	37	M	6.6	7.7	85	1.85	3.5	TN	
161	30	M	9.0	8.6	104	1.82	4.9	TN	
163	55	M	6.2	6.7	93	1.92	3.2	TN	
165	49	M	8.1	7.9	103	1.92	4.2	TN	
166	40	M	8.2	7.8	105	1.92	4.3	TN	
167	33	M	10.1	9.3	108	1.78	5.7	TN	
171	37	M	5.5	7.7	71	1.58	3.5	FP	

ID	=	identification number
D	=	determined
P	=	predicted cardiac output in liters/min
SA	=	surface area of the body in m^2
CI	=	cardiac index
PRED	=	prediction
TN	=	true negative
FN	=	false negative
TP	=	true positive
FP	=	false positive

TABLE F-3. Subjects with Subsequent Myocardial Infarction

N=28

ID	DATE	AGE SEX D	P	D/P	SA	CI	PRED.	COMMENTS
002	12. 3.66	68 M 5.7	9.0	63	1.90	3.0	TP*	
	2.13.67	Sudden Death						
003	1. 5.63	65 M 5.0	6.8	73	1.97	2.5	FP	
	3.37.64	Sudden Death						
005	6. 3.63	66 M 3.8	5.6	68	1.90	2.0	TP*	
	7. 8.63	Sudden Death						
006	4. 1.67	66 F 4.1	5.4	77	1.48	2.8	FP	
	3.10.68	Sudden Death						
008	1. 5.63	59 M 5.6	7.8	71	2.05	2.7	FP	
	8. 9.64	Sudden Death						
013	12.21.64	68 M 4.9	5.3	93	1.80	2.7	FN*	
	4.29.65	Fatal MI						
014	3.20.65	48 M 6.2	6.7	93	1.62	3.8	FN*	
	6.29.65	Non-fatal MI						
016	1.19.63	74 F 5.2	6.5	80	1.54	3.4	TN	
	1.28.65	Non-fatal MI						
	11.22.67	2.3	6.2	37	1.40	1.6	TP*	
	1. 6.68	Sudden Death						
017	3.23.65	70 F 3.6	6.1	58	1.71	2.1	TP*	
	9. 4.65	Fatal MI						
018	12.18.64	73 F 3.6	7.8	46	1.53	2.4	TP*	
	1.15.65	Sudden Death						
020	5.12.62	50 M 5.0	7.8	64	1.93	2.6	FP	
	2. 3.64	Non-fatal MI						
	7.28.65	4.9	6.5	74	1.98	2.5	TP*	
	8.12.65	Non-fatal MI						
	5.14.66	5.3	6.5	81	1.98	2.6	FN*	
	7. 4.66	Fatal MI						
031	3.20.65	36 M 7.3	9.4	78	1.95	3.7	TP*	
	6.22.65	Non-fatal MI						
	7. 6.65	9.7	9.3	105	1.98	4.9	TN	Still hospitalized
	3.28.66	Fatal MI						
034	9.22.62	51 M 4.5	6.4	70	1.74	2.7	TP*	
	10.31.62	Non-fatal MI						
	1.29.66	4.3	6.7	65	1.74	2.7	TP*	
	1.29.66	Non-fatal MI, some hours after test						
	2.11.66	4.8	6.2	77	1.75	2.7	TP*	
	2.23.66	Non-fatal MI						
035	6.18.66	37 F 6.2	8.1	76	1.68	3.7	TP*	
	11.30.66	Fatal MI						
043	1.12.63	61 M 5.7	7.0	81	1.93	3.0	TN	
	5.31.64	Sudden Death						
048	2.12.66	54 M 7.6	8.0	99	2.04	3.7	FN*	
	7.20.66	Non-fatal MI						
050	1. 8.65	65. F 5.7	7.1	80	1.59	3.6	FN*	
	1.16.65	Fatal MI						
052	4.14.67	49 M 9.3	9.3	100	2.02	4.6	TN	
	2. 6.68	Non-fatal MI						

TABLE F-3. (continued)

N=28

ID	DATE	AGE	SEX	D	P	D/P	SA	CI	PRED.	COMMENTS
054	12.27.67	63	M	5.4	7.1	76	1.93	2.6	TP*	
	1.16.68			3.6	8.8	41	Non-fatal MI same day, angina during test			
	2. 3.68			5.3	6.5	82	2.08	2.6	TN	Still in hospital
	8.21.68	Fatal MI								
055	5.15.63	57	M	6.0	7.3	82	1.76	3.4	FN*	
	7.25.63	Sudden Death								
058	4.10.65	83	F	2.9	4.5	65	1.30	2.2	TP*	
	8.13.65	Sudden Death								
063	2.11.67	63	M	10.1	7.8	129	1.97	5.1	FN*	Alcohol intoxicated
	4.27.67	Non-fatal MI								
072	8.20.66	62	M	6.3	8.8	71	2.04	3.1	TP*	Originally a control
	9. ·· .66	Silent MI								
078	11.13.65	47	M	7.9	8.0	99	1.79	4.4	TN	
	6. 6.66	Sudden Death								
079	1. 2.65	38	M	6.6	7.8	84	1.92	3.4	TN	
	7.23.65	Fatal MI								
086	3. 5.66	45	M	7.5	8.2	92	1.85	4.0	FN*	Hypertension
	3.22.66	Non-fatal MI								
	3.31.66			6.7	8.5	79	1.90	3.5	TP*	Still in hospital
	4. 8.66	Sudden Death, Hemorrhage into the left circumflex cor. art. intima.								
094	12.16.64	64	M	8.7	9.0	96	1.92	4.5	TN	
	2.22.67	Sudden Death								
099	6.10.63	67	M	5.7	8.9	64	1.98	2.9	FP	
	2. 4.64	Sudden Death								

*Within six months.

ID	=	identification number
D	=	determined
P	=	predicted cardiac output in liters/min
SA	=	surface area of the body in m^2
CI	=	cardiac index
PRED	=	prediction
TN	=	true negative
FN	=	false negative
TP	=	true positive
FP	=	false positive

There were 94 cardiac outputs above 80% which were not followed by an infarction within six months of assessment, but there were eight which were. The risk of myocardial infarction or sudden death within six months after a normal hemodynamic assessment is therefore:

$$\frac{\text{FALSE NEGATIVE}}{\text{TRUE NEGATIVE} + \text{FALSE NEGATIVE}} = \frac{8}{94 + 8} = 7\%$$

Twenty-two individuals who had hemodynamic assessments suffered a myocardial infarction or sudden death within six months of their assessment. Fifteen of these were below 80% and seven were normal. The risk of having a myocardial infarction or suffering sudden death shortly after an abnormal hemodynamic assessment is therefore:

159

$$\frac{\text{TRUE POSITIVE}}{\text{TRUEPOSITIVE} + \text{FALSEPOSITIVE}} = \frac{15}{15 + 7} = 68\%$$

The results are plotted graphically in Figure F-10. It is interesting to note that several of the false positives were followed by myocardial infarctions which occurred later than six months after evaluation and several false negatives were close to the lower limit of 80%. One false negative evaluation is worthy of note since it was a high value, but this patient (063) was intoxicated by alcohol at the time of the test.

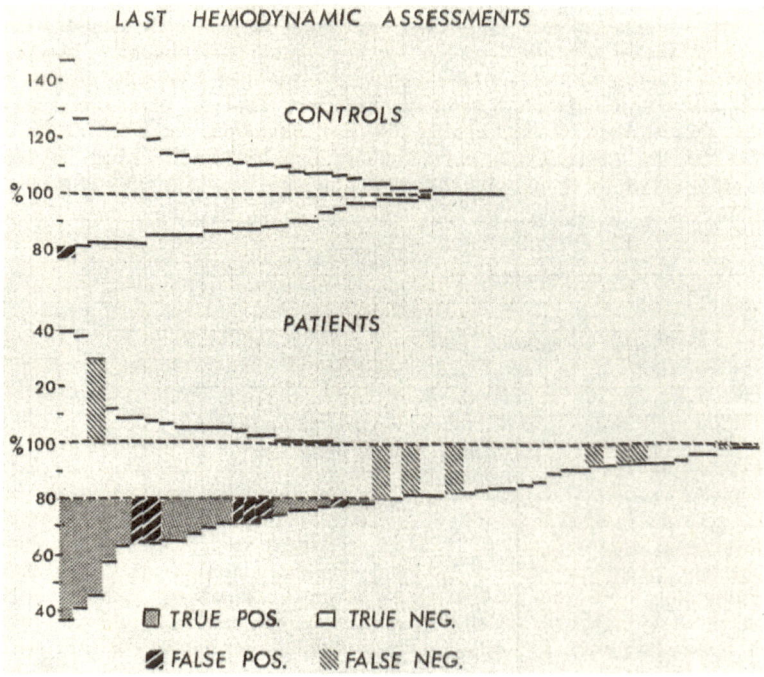

FIG. F-10. Distribution of hemodynamic assessment. Distribution around 100%. Only last hemodynamic assessment and the one preceding each myocardial infarction or sudden death are marked. Patients 016, 031 and 086 are listed twice, 020, 034, and 054 three times, corresponding to each of their infarctions. The mycoardial infarction on 1/16/68 of patient 054 is listed both before and also at the actual time of the event. Note symmetrical distribution (98% within normal limits of 100 ± 20%) among the controls and skewed distribution among patients. The majority of the assessments below 80% lead to a myocardial infarction or sudden death and most of these events occur within six months; the three lowest, within six weeks.

Only one control (072) had a myocardial infarction during the study. The prediction for this event was positive, and there is no evidence to suggest that the mechanism of myocardial infarction in this control was any different from that in patients; however, data are too few to generalize this conclusion. Even when the prediction period was extended or when patients only were included in the computations, the accuracy for negative predictions remained essentially unchanged, but in such manipulations the percentage of false positives increased.

Half the subjects in this study had had a myocardial infarction prior to entering the study and, therefore, constituted a high-risk group. This explains the high rate of recurrent infarctions in the patient group. However, it does not explain why myocardial infarctions or sudden deaths occurred within the predicted time frame when cardiac output was low but not when it was normal. The chance for incident should have been equal at either low or normal cardiac output, since the outputs were very variable and each subject was represented equally in the computation of risk. A prediction rate of 68% for myocardial infarction or sudden death within six months, with only a false positive prediction of 7%, suggests that low cardiac output is indeed a precipitating factor. However, since several normal cardiac outputs were recorded shortly before an infarction, one is led to the conclusion that low cardiac output is not the only factor involved. Perhaps, physiological shifts change the hemodynamic assessment picture frequently within a six-month period.

Predictive value is claimed for the Master's "2-step" exercise test. The claim is based on a threefold increase in myocardial infarctions or sudden death in patients with specified electrocardiographic changes, assuming a normal death rate in such subjects of about three per thousand. Table F-4 lists the distribution of positive and negative results from five commonly quoted studies. The test was positive in 25% of these populations, yet 80% of these positive predictions turned out to be false in the subsequent four, five, and ten-year followup regardless of whether a previous infarction existed or not.

Great efforts are presently being made to define factors predisposing to myocardial infarction. The results of this study suggest that a low cardiac output, and the presumed concomitant sluggish blood flow, may produce intravascular thromboses in the coronary vessels. If diminished cardiac output can be explained on the basis of myocardial inotropic activity, it might be possible to explain, through a single mechanism, the greater tendency toward myocardial infarction noted in conditions requiring more work from the heart, such as stress, obesity, hypertension, emphysema, or those conditions which decrease the fatigue resistance of heart muscle, such as sedentary work, age, or previous valvular, myocardial, or coronary disease. The slow flow rate concomitant with decreased cardiac output might at the same time explain the increased tendency for intravascular thromboses to form in narrowed arteriosclerotic vessels commonly present in cases of advanced age, diabetes, and high blood cholesterol. If such a hypothesis should be correct, studies of these different predisposing factors will have to be conducted while measuring cardiac output or else it will be very difficult to achieve meaningful data.

Intriguing possibilities for therapy emerge from consideration of this study. Since low cardiac output is singled out as a main precipitating factor in myocardial infarction, increasing cardiac output seems like a rational approach towards preventing myocardial infarction. The condition of low cardiac output was observed to be· reversible, often returning to normal shortly after an acute infarction, and much faster than can be expected from a healing process. Such a phenomenon is not incompatible with a theory of inotropic etiology as a cause for low cardiac output. If such a theory can be supported, it might well be the most important finding in this study. If normal cardiac output represents a low-risk condition, then increasing cardiac output to normal by means of rest and medical management might represent a preventive or "postponing" program. A hemodynamic assessment below 80% should, therefore, initiate medical management to increase stroke volume and lower circulating blood volume.

Suggesting radiocardiograms for routine screening and preventive medicine raises the question of the advisability of exposing a seemingly normal person to an invasive, radioactive procedure. Technically, the patient is only subjected to a laboratory procedure which is routinely used for the determination of serum blood volume, and the technique has an outstanding safety record. The author has personally performed close to 5,000 determinations and has never observed any ill effects.

Radiocardiograms require about 10 to 15µCi of ^{131}I human serum albumin. This will expose the patient to a radiation dose of about 20% of that which he would receive in a routine chest x-ray which is about 30 mrad.[29] From a radiation safety viewpoint, therefore, indications for the procedure can be rather wide. Clinical considerations as to when to use the technique and how much time to allow between followups should depend upon the specific risk factors present in each patient. The patients in this study were seen from one to three times

TABLE F-4. Predictive Value for the Master's 2-Step Exercise Test

	TOTAL Tot.	POSITIVES Tot.	%	True	%	False	%	NEGATIVES Tot.	%	True	%	False	%	COMMENTS
Diamond[7]	153	37	21	16	43	21	57	116	76	100	86	16	14	Railway employees with known or suspected cor. disease. Five year follow-up.
Franco[8]	544	135	25	16	12	119	88	409	75	403	98	6	2	Periodic health exam. Ten year follow-up.
Mattingly[9]	871	145	17	40	28	105	73	726	83	708	98	18	2	Periodic health exam. Ten year follow-up.
Brody[10]	756	280	37	32	11	248	89	476	62	456	96	20	4	Periodic health exam. in business executives. Mean follow-up 4 years.
Robb[11]	1373	269	20	27	9	242	91	861	62	845	98	16	2	Life insurance exam. Mean follow-up 5 years. Mixed medical indications.
Rob[11]	265	84	32 X̄25	15	18 X̄20	69	82 X̄80	181	68 X̄71	174	96 X̄95	7	4 X̄5	Life insurance exam. Mean follow-up 5 years. Pat. with known cor. disease.
This study	126	22	18	15	68	7	32	102	82	93	91	9	9	Total number is different from number of patients because some patients had several infarctions.

163

each year, with those considered as higher risks being seen more frequently. Although some patients displayed fast changes in their hemodynamic assessment and some changes might have been missed, it appears that in general a conservative program can be successful. Few patients should need a test more often than every four months, and any who do should be in the very high-risk category. Future experience will, no doubt, further define the most effective program.

SUMMARY

Radiocardiograms proved to be a practical, reproducible, and highly accurate procedure for measuring cardiac output. The clinical assessment of cardiac output, using the cardiac index method, was found to be misleading and mathematically invalid. Clinical hemodynamic assessment can only be obtained by predicting cardiac output from a multiple regression formula which includes factors for age, pulse, and blood volume, and then computing the percent difference between the determined cardiac output and the predicted cardiac output. The percent difference is called hemodynamic assessment because it expresses the efficiency with which a heart pumps the body's circulating blood volume. Low hemodynamic assessments preceded myocardial infarctions or sudden death so often within six months after the determination that it was undeniably of predictive value. A low hemodynamic assessment suggested that a measurable, but pre symptomatic heart failure with concomitant sluggish bloodstream is present, and represents a high-risk state. These assessments also suggest that a therapeutic program, directed toward increasing stroke volume and decreasing circulating blood volume, might be the best regimen to prescribe for the patient at high risk in regard to myocardial infarction.

Acknowledgement

The author wishes to express his gratitude to all of his colleagues and the staff of the Neurocardiology Research Center. Doctors Stewart G. Wolf, Director; C.G. Gunn, Administrator; E.N. Brandt, study design and statistical analysis; R. Duncan, study design and statistical analysis; R. Schneider, autonomic responses; M.E. Groover, Jr., blood protein analysis; J. Naughton, exercise physiology; J.W. Hampton, coagulation research; H. Wulff, fat and carbohydrate metabolism; T.N. Lynn, electrocardiograph and ballistocardiograph; J. Kalbfleisch, electrocardiography, coronary catheterization; C.W. Smith, catecholamine determinations; C. Dubowsky, blood chemistry; P. Houk, diving reflex, heart catheterization; C.A. Adsett, psychiatric interviews; A. Paredes, psychiatric interviews; J.O. Bruhn, sociological interviews; A.M. Modkoff, psychological interviews, and Miss L. Boone, dietetic interviews.

It was seven years of the most stimulating research. Nothing reported here could have been accomplished without the dedicated efforts of all the other investigators.

I express gratitude to Mrs. Elaine Patrick, my technician, who carried out all procedures with meticulous care.

With the greatest of respect are also remembered the more than 100 volunteers who visited our 8:00 Saturday morning clinic every six weeks for up to seven years—their only motivation being that their effort might contribute something to medical science. None of the professional members of this study can match this contribution.

Finally, I wish to extend my thanks to Dr. Seymour N. Stein, Chief, Medical Office, NASA-Ames Research Center. It was a privilege for me to have Dr. Stein edit both Parts I and II before submitting them for publication.

Gunnar Sevelius, MD

DISCUSSION

Dr. Hoffer (University of Chicago): Dr. Sevelius, as I understand it, all of your patients whom you studied were patients who had had previous myocardial infarctions and had them prior to the initiation of the study.

Dr. Sevelius: No, half of them.

Dr. Hoffer: I'm wondering if the 58 patients who had had myocardial infarctions might in fact have a low cardiac output predicated on the basis of the extent of their infarction and you are really measuring the extent of the infarction rather than actually making a valid prediction that the decrease in the cardiac output is responsible for their reinfarction. Maybe you have to go to a normal control group before you can really make any sort of predictive statement about the value of the cardiac output in predicting myocardial infarction in a normal population. I am trying to say that both the reinfarction and decrease in cardiac output may in fact just be manifestations of the underlying cardiac disease rather than the underlying disease in fact being decreased cardiac output.

Dr. Sevelius: We measured the cardiac output at the beginning and you saw it coming down. When it was low, they had their heart attacks. In those who did not die, cardiac output often returned to normal faster than any healing process could explain. In one patient this repeated itself three times. I agree, if you have a previous heart attack, you are more apt to have a low cardiac output. Your fatigue resistance in the heart muscle is less, so the variability and the lower dip were more common in the group with previous coronary disease. This was very likely due to their predisposing condition. I feel the results of the study suggest that low cardiac output, with accompanying slow blood flow, might be a precipitating factor causing the intravascular thrombosis which leads to the myocardial infarction.

Dr. Hoffer: It would seem to me that measuring the cardiac output would be a good predictive test possibly of indexing those patients who have had a previous myocardial infarction. It may be an index which may be helpful in predicting reinfarction. But, I'm just wondering if you can extrapolate this information to normal population.

Dr. Sevelius: No, I cannot. That's why I said you can only apply our results to our population. It was a high-risk population which we studied. I expect, however, that predictions would not be less accurate in normal population because it is easier to be accurate in a population with a high percentage of true normals. It is more difficult to work with an already diseased population because they are apt to give you many true and false positive results. If you have had a heart attack, you will not necessarily have another one within six months. The chance of having a second heart attack is about ten times greater than to have a first one, or about 3%, without a time limit set on when the second will occur. We are saying that you have a 70% chance to have a second heart attack within six months, when your cardiac output is low. The difference is that low cardiac output then pinpoints the high-risk period, so that preventive measures can be started before anatomical changes have occurred. As you know, a cardiac output which is low from inotropic fatigue can easily be corrected.

Dr. Goodun (Saint Francis Hospital, Tulsa): I was wondering what interest you or anyone else in the group might have in peripheral blood flow. Your study seems to be excellent for this purpose. You might place external monitors in other positions, such as the carotids, the iliacs, the popliteals, and so forth and assess peripheral blood flow at the same time as you measure cardiac output. Is there any interest here?

Dr. Sevelius: Yes, I think there is great interest in trying to develop peripheral blood flow measurements quantitatively. Several attempts have been made that are promising, but the mathematics and physics involved in determining branched flow get very involved.

Dr. Goodun: If you have symmetrically located detectors placed over symmetrical organs, why would you need to quantitate; why not just qualitate?

Dr. Sevelius: Yes, you might qualitate or make a comparative estimate. For the femoral arteries, for instance, the peak heights of two flow curves recorded over each femoral and divided by their equilibriums would yield a good comparative measurement for the flow in each artery. You cannot express it in milliliters, but you can say it in a ratio if you use the peak of the flow curve and divide it with its equilibrium. It will correlate linearly with the flow in the branch up to about 12% of the cardiac output, and very few arteries have any greater blood flow than this.

REFERENCES

1. Sevelius, G., Cardiac output. *In* Sevelius, G., ed. Radioisotopes and Circulation. Little, Brown and Co., Boston, 1965, p. 118.

2. Nadler, S.B. and Hidalgo, J.U. Blood volume. *In* Sevelius, G., ed. Radioisotopes and Circulation. Little, Brown and Co., Boston, 1965, p. 65.

3. Powers, J.E. and Sevelius, G. Fundamentals of data interpretation. *In* Sevelius, G., ed. Radioisotopes and Circulation. Little, Brown and Co., Boston, 1965, p. 25.

4. Huff, R.L., Feller, D.D. and Bogardus, G. Cardiac output by body surface counting of I-131 human serum albumin. *J. Clin. Invest.*, 33:944, 1954.

5. Van der Feer, Y. Cardiac output measured by injection method without arterial sampling. *Amer. Heart J.,* 56:642, 1958.

6. Veal, N. and Vetter, H. Radioisotope Techniques in Clinical Research and Diagnosis. Butterworth & Co., London, 1958.

7. Shackman, R. Radioactive isotope measurement of cardiac output. *Clin. Sci.*, 17:317, 1958.

8. Pritchard, W.H., MacIntyre, W.J. and Moir, T.W. The determination of cardiac output by dilution method without arterial sampling. *J. Lab. Clin. Med.*, 46:939, 1955.

9. Schreiner, B.F., Jr., Yu, P.D. and Lovejoy, F.W. Estimation of cardiac output from precordial dilution curves in patients with cardiopulmonary disease. *Circ. Res.*, 7:595, 1959.

10. Zeckert, H.F., Herbig, F. and Cooper, T. Serial determination of cardiac output from precordial isotope dilution curves. *J. Nucl. Med.*, 7:424, 1966.

11. Kloster, E.F., Bristown, D.J. and Griswold, H.E. Cardiac output determination from precordial isotope-dilution curves during exercise. *J. Appl. Phys.*, 465:26, 1969.

12. Guyton, A.C. and Coleman, G.T. Long term regulation of the circulation: interrelationships with body fluid volumes. *In* Reeves, E.B. and Guyton, A.C., eds. Physical Basis of Circulatory Transport: Regulation and Exchange. W.B. Saunders Co., Philadelphia, 1967, p. 200.

13. Tanner, J.M. Fallacy of per weight and per surface area standards and their relation to previous correlations. *J. Appl. Physiol.*, 2:1, 1949.

14. Taylor, H.L. and Tiede, K. A comparison of the estimation of the basal cardiac output from a linear formula and the cardiac index. *J. Clin. Invest.*, 31:209, 1952.

15. Smulyan, H., Vincent, W.A., Kosenesout, D., Cuddy, R.P., and Eich, R.H. An evaluation of the cardiac index. *Amer. Heart J.*, 72:621, 1966.

16. Sevelius, G., and Modica, G. Valori normali di portata cardiaco (metodo radiocardiografico): Proposta di una formula personale per la espressione corretta dell'indice cardiaco. *Atti Soc Ital di Cardiologia*, 2:93, 1964.

17. National Academy of Sciences, National Research Council. Handbook of Circulation. W.B. Saunders Co., Philadelphia, 1950.

18. Smith, W.W., Wikler, N.S. and Fox, A.C. Hemodynamic studies of patients with myocardial infarction. *Circulation*, 9:352, 1954.

19. Malmcrona, R. and Varnauskas, E. Hemodynamics in acute myocardial infarction. *Acta Med. Scand.*, 175:fasc. 1, 1964.

20. Thomas, M., Malmcrona, R., and Shillingford, J.P. Hemodynamic changes in patients with acute myocardial infarction. *Circulation*, 31:811, 1965.

21. Freis, E.D., Schnaper, H.W., Johnson, R.L. and Schreiner, G.E. Hemodynamic alterations in acute myocardial infarction. I. Cardiac output, mean arterial pressure, total blood volumes, venous pressure, and average circulation time. *J. Clin. Invest.*, 31: 131, 1952.

22. Murphy, G.W., Glick, G., Schreiner, B.F. and Yu, P.D. Cardiac output in acute myocardial infarction. *Amer. J. Cardiol.*, 11:587, 1963.

23. Wolf, S.G. Psychosocial forces in myocardial infarction and sudden death. *Circulation*, 40, Suppl., 4:74, 1969.

24. Dimond, G. The exercise test and prognosis of coronary heart disease. *Circulation*, 24:736, 1961.

25. Franco, S.C., Gerl, A.J., and Murphy, G.T. Periodic health examinations: A long term study 1949-1959. *J. Occup. Med.*, 3:13, 1961.

26. Mattingly, T.W. The postexercise electrocardiogram. Its value in the diagnosis and prognosis of coronary arterial disease. *Amer. J. Cardiol.*, 9:395, 1962.

27. Brody, A.J. Master's "2-step" exercise test in clinically unselected patients. *J.A.M.A.*, 171:1195, 1959.

28. Robb, G.P. and Marks, H.H. Latent coronary artery disease. Determination of its presence and severity by the exercise electrocardiogram. *Amer. J. Cardiol.*, 13:603, 1964.

29. Loevinger, R., Holt, J.G. and Hine, G.J. Internally administered radioisotopes. *In* Hine, G.J., and Brownell, G.L., eds. Radiation Dosimetry. Academic Press, Inc., New York, 1956.

www.ingramcontent.com/pod-product-compliance
Lightning Source LLC
Chambersburg PA
CBHW020419290526
45785CB00002B/641